PSYCHOSOCIAL DIMENSIONS OF THE
OF THE
PREGNANT FAMILY

Laurie Nehls Sherwen, Ph.D., R.N., is Project Director of the Maternal-Infant Core Competency Project, a three-year federally funded project housed at the March of Dimes Birth Defects Foundation in White Plains, New York. Prior to her current position, she was an assistant professor and coordinator of the Graduate Parent-Child Nursing Program at Rutgers, The State University, College of Nursing, where she wrote and received funding for the Perinatal Track Grant. Dr. Sherwen received her B.S.N. from Seton Hall University, and her M.A. and Ph.D. from New York University. She is author, co-author, and editor of numerous articles and books concerned with pregnancy and parenting, including *Analysis and Application of Nursing Research: Parent-Neonate Studies,* which received an American Journal of Nursing Book of the Year Award in 1984. She has done research in the areas of psychological states of expectant mothers and fathers, and bonding between mothers and adopted children.

Psychosocial Dimensions of the Pregnant Family

Laurie Nehls ⎫Sherwen, Ph.D., R.N.

with contributors

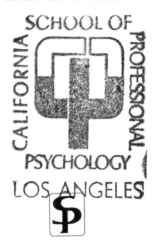

Springer Publishing Company
New York

This book is dedicated to Dorothy W. Smith, Ed.D., R.N., who was a mentor, long before it was fashionable.

Springer Publishing Company, Inc.
536 Broadway
New York, NY 10012

87 88 89 90 91 / 5 4 3 2 1

Printed in the United States of America

Library of Congress Cataloging-in-Publication Data

Sherwen, Laurie Nehls, 1947–
    Psychosocial dimensions of the pregnant family.

    Includes bibliographies and index.
    1. Pregnancy—Psychological aspects. 2. Pregnancy—
Social aspects. 3. Pregnant women—Family relationships.
4. Obstetrical nursing. I. Title. [DNLM: 1. Family—
nurses' instruction. 2. Obstetrical Nursing.
3. Pregnancy—nurses' instruction. WY 157 S554p]
RG560.S48   1986   618.2′0019   86-28027
ISBN 0-8261-4380-1

Contents

Contributing Authors

Cynthia B. Hughes, Ed.D., R.N.C., Associate Professor, Graduate Department, Seton Hall University, South Orange, New Jersey

Jeanne Toussie Jacobwitz, M.S.N., M.P.H., C.N.M., Morristown Memorial Hospital, Morristown, New Jersey

Susan Kutzner, Ph.D., R.N., Assistant Professor of Nursing, The University of Rhode Island, College of Nursing, Kingston, Rhode Island; and Senior Planner, Commonwealth of Massachusetts, Department of Public Health, Division of Family Health Services, Maternal-Child Health, Boston, Massachusetts

Ellen Schuzman, M.A., R.N., Assistant Professor of Nursing, Rutgers, The State University, College of Nursing, Newark, New Jersey

Carol Toussie-Weingarten, Ph.D., R.N., Villanova University, College of Nursing, Philadelphia, Pennsylvania; and Nursing Research Consultant, Parent Project, Morristown Memorial Hospital, Morristown, New Jersey

Acknowledgments

I would like to acknowledge some individuals whose help, support, and encouragement were essential to my efforts. First and foremost are my past and present graduate students, whose ideas, challenges, and insights helped me to refine my own ideas concerning the pregnant family. I hope they learned near as much from me as I did from them.

For her belief in my abilities and encouragement when I doubted them, I thank Carol Toussie-Weingarten, colleague and long-time friend. I thank my former colleagues and friends at Rutgers College of Nursing for their interest in this work and their input into my conceptualization of the childbearing family. My appreciation goes to Ruth Chasek of Springer Publishing Company for her critique and support of this work. Also, thanks to Janice Brzozowski and Doreen Formisano for typing the manuscript. Finally, thanks to my husband, Doug, my greatest critic and fan, for his undying sense of humor and appreciation of the absurd.

LAURIE NEHLS SHERWEN

Introduction

The preparation of this book stems from my role as teacher of parent-child clinical nurse specialists. Along with many of my colleagues, I have been acutely aware of a lack of organized content in nursing concerning psychosocial aspects of individuals and families during pregnancy. This book represents what I would have liked to have had available in teaching my graduate students. It provides a starting point for nurses wanting to delve more deeply into issues concerning the psychosocial aspects of the pregnant family. It is hoped that it will stimulate thinking and questioning in the reader and provide an impetus for empirical inquiry into this underresearched area.

As students in a parent-child nursing masters program in the early 1970s, my colleagues and I were often faced with the question, "What on earth can a nurse with a masters degree do during a pregnancy?" At the time, pregnancy was viewed as a basically healthy state and "Lamaze" childbirth preparation was coming into its own. The focus on "pregnancy and health" denied us the forms of advanced interventions open to students in the course offering a masters degree in medical/surgical nursing. The baccalaureate nurse had all the qualifications necessary to handle nursing care of the woman during the prenatal period, labor and delivery, and puerperium. In fact, many of us were put to shame in our skills by 20-year veterans of the labor and delivery suites. And the intended role for students enrolled in midwifery masters programs was obviously the psychological and physiological management of low-risk pregnancy, labor and delivery, and the puerperium. For us, however, there was no clear-cut role to move into when working with pregnant women on an "advanced" level. We obviously had to chart new ground and clarify our nursing role and interventions.

We were fortunate as students at New York University to have two professors who had a handle on what a masters-prepared parent-child nurse should do. Drs. Luz Porter and Mary Guiffra had the vision, before general acceptance of the Clinical Nurse Specialist, to define an appropriate role for the advanced practitioner in maternity nursing. The focus of our interventions actually had two dimensions, the first less revolutionary than the second. As undergraduates, we were aware that there was a psychological aspect to the woman's evolving pregnancy and giving birth. As masters' students we became aware of the psychosocial dimensions of pregnancy in great depth, not only in the mother but also in the father and siblings. Perhaps more unusual at that time was the concept that the *family* was actually "pregnant," and that the pregnant family, as a whole, was our client. In the early 1970s, systems theory as a form of family therapy was not so widespread, especially as a theory used in nursing. Thus, we had to reorient our thinking and look not just at a pregnant woman with a family, but at a family who shared the pregnancy experience in a dynamic manner. Pregnancy truly affects all parts of the family system. The answer to our question was slowly forthcoming: Being an advanced practitioner of parent-child nursing in the maternity realm meant working with the *entire* childbearing family and focusing in particular on the psychosocial dynamics that form family interactions.

This book represents one answer to the question, "What does the parent-child clinical nurse specialist need to know to fulfill an advanced role with the pregnant client?" This answer has served me well in the teaching of masters degree students and it has served my students well when, as practitioners, they have carved a niche for themselves in a maternity setting.

OVERVIEW OF CHAPTERS

Chapter 1 provides an overview and review of some variables of importance in assessing family dynamics, and it provides a glossary of systems theory terms. The reader very familiar with family theory may skip this chapter without affecting comprehension of subsequent chapters.

Chapter 2 examines the family system specifically during pregnancy and discusses the tasks and transitions that occur in some of its dynamics and subsystems. Crisis is suggested as a model for nursing intervention with the pregnant family.

An important aspect of working with the pregnant family is assessment of the family system. Chapter 3 looks at the manner and methodologies by which the nurse may assess the pregnant family system.

Chapter 4 looks at sexuality in the pregnant family system—not just in terms of sexual function during pregnancy but also in terms of sexual structures that give rise to function. The concepts of sex roles and androgyny in the pregnant family are discussed.

Chapters 5, 6, and 7 discuss the pregnant woman as an individual system within the broader family unit. Such psychosocial dimensions as the process of maternal role attainment, fantasy patterns during pregnancy, and evolution of the body image during pregnancy are explored.

Chapters 8 and 9 examine psychosocial changes that occur in other members of the pregnant family, namely, the father and siblings of the infant-to-be. As with all previous chapters, nursing interventions are suggested that will facilitate resolution of health deviations in the family or individual dynamics.

Chapters 10 and 11 look at some trends in modes of birthing, in types of caretakers available to the pregnant family, in government and private health care systems, and in nursing research during the childbearing phase. Some major issues surrounding delivery of care to the pregnant family are identified.

This book draws together research and theories from many disciplines concerning psychosocial dimensions of the childbearing family. It is hoped that it will not only suggest new aspects of nursing interventions with these families but also stimulate the readers to discover for themselves additional dimensions of the pregnant family.

Chapter 1

A General Introduction To Family Structure and Function

This book is based on the concept that each family functions as a system of interacting parts. When a woman becomes pregnant, that condition affects the other members of her family. For this reason, the entire family can be said to share in the pregnancy; hence we have adopted a term that will be used throughout the book—*the pregnant family*. While individual members of the pregnant family must be assessed for their responses to the pregnancy, understanding how their behaviors are parts of a larger unit, the family, is important. These family behaviors will incorporate individual responses but will be unique, based on the dynamic interactions that occur between individuals with different backgrounds, perceptions, and feelings about the pregnancy. Interpretation of behaviors and design of nursing interventions will be different depending on whether it is the family system or the individual components of that system that are observed. Therefore, this chapter focuses on variables that are important in families in general and presents a basis for understanding changes that will occur in these variables during pregnancy. To aid the reader in understanding systems theory as a branch of family theory, a glossary of systems terms is included as a reference at the back of the chapter.

DEFINITIONS OF THE FAMILY SYSTEM

The concept of family system used in this book is an adaptation of the concept developed by psychology and psychiatry. In these disciplines, family systems theory arose from the so-called "family movement," which began in the early and mid 1950s. Bowen (1978) describes the origin of the movement as an attempt to provide better treatment for complex emotional problems not amenable to traditional individual-oriented therapies built on the medical model.

Bowen further indicates that there are many ways to view the family. He gives impetus to the view of family as a system since "a change in one part of the system is followed by compensatory change in other parts of the system" (1978, p.187). The family system, to Bowen, is composed of a variety of systems and subsystems that function at all levels of efficiency, from optimum functioning to total dysfunction and failure. Further, the functioning of the family system, as with any system, is dependent on the functioning of both its subsystems and the larger systems of which it is a part. Some of the main functional patterns observed in families have been formulated into component concepts that comprise current family theory, of which family systems theory is a branch.

Sedgewick (1978), a nurse, also finds the concept of family as system a useful framework for psychiatric nursing. She defines a family as "an integrated system of interdependent structures and functions, [which] is constituted of relationships, and consists of people who must learn to live together" (p.31). Patterns of behavior are referred to as *components* or *units;* in combination with other components, they interrelate to produce the overall system known as the family. In essence, the family is a network or system of relationships.

Friedman (1978), also a nurse, defines family as a living social system, a small group of closely interrelated and interdependent individuals who are organized into a single unit so as to attain a specific purpose, namely, the family functions or goals. Friedman, seeing the family as the appropriate framework for community nursing, states that the interrelationships that are found in a family system are so intricately tied together that a change in any one part inevitably results in changes in the entire system.

Thus, from several perspectives, it seems highly useful to view the family from a systems viewpoint. Systems theory gives a reasonable framework for analyzing what goes on within the family, as well as the family's interactions with those units external to it. In addition, a systems framework prescribes interventions for complex problems related to family health and well-being, considering the family as a whole. Following this train of thought, Beavers (1977), a psychiatrist, gives an excellent theoretical construct for viewing family function and wellness. Such a model may be of great use in nursing, where the concern is wellness across the mind–body continuum of an individual or group. The following model also is useful in consideration of the childbearing family, where concepts of crisis and stress are sure to impinge on the unit.

A THEORETICAL MODEL FOR VIEWING THE FAMILY SYSTEM

Beavers (1977) very simply proposes a continuum by which to order families with respect to effectiveness or, in nursing terms, level of well-

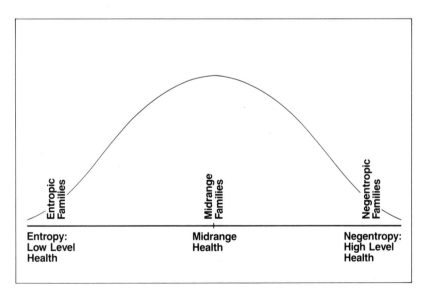

Figure 1-1. Continuum of Family Level of Health

ness. At one end of the continuum are the most flexible, adaptable, goal-achieving family systems (i.e., negentropic families). At the other end of the continuum are the most inflexible, undifferentiated, and ineffective systems (i.e., entropic families).

Sherwen (1981) has proposed a similar model, shown in schematic form in Figure 1–1. This schematic representation includes the concept of the "normal curve" and implies that the majority of families are neither totally negentropic nor entropic, but somewhere in between. Nursing intervention for the family, then, would include, as a goal, assisting the family to achieve a higher level of negentropy, that is, complexity, organization, differentiation, control, and flexibility. Such attributes are hallmarks of a healthy family system in both a physical and psychological sense.

VARIABLES OF IMPORTANCE IN THE FAMILY SYSTEM

Different family systems theorists focus on different family variables as important in understanding the way a family functions. Several of these variables will be considered.

Structure

Several different concepts are subsumed into the variable of structure. The first is that of the *family subsystem*. Friedman (1981) describes these subsystems as being made up of sets of relationships involving two or more family members, often having different levels of power. Depending upon the nature of the family—for example, the nuclear family or extended family—several of these interpersonal subsystems are inherent in a family. There is the *spouse subsystem,* where two adult members relate to each other as marital partners and parents of offspring. Closely related to this subsystem is the concept of *parental coalition,* which indicates the strength or weakness of the parents' ability to work together and to lead the family effectively (Beavers, 1977).

Another common one is the *parent-child subsystem,* composed of parents and their children. A third is the *sibling subsystem,* indicating the family's children's relationships with each other. Other subsystems that may exist in a family involve relationships between nuclear family members and extended family members, such as the *grandparent-*

grandchild subsystem. These subsystems take on great importance in considering the concept of family networks.

Another vital concept that may be included under the variable of family system structure is that of the *triangle.* This concept is discussed by Bowen (1978) and has great import for understanding the changes in family structure that occur with childbirth. Bowen sees the family system as made up of a variety of subsystems that constantly interact and repattern, depending on the state of the family system and its interactions with its environment. In calm periods, two members have a comfortable emotional alliance (form a dyad). A third member moves in and gains the favor of one member (or is rejected) and thus sets up tension within the system. The tension, in turn, sets up emotional circuits that spread to all other subsystems or interlocking triangles in a system, causing large-scale repatterning to occur. A triangle is traditionally seen as a subsystem of two interacting individuals and one isolate; thus it can be very unstable and can set up great negative affect in the family system.

Another important family concept that is often considered as part of the structure is that of *closeness.* This involves both the clarity of subsystem boundaries and also the amount of sharing and intimacy evidenced in the family interaction (Beavers, 1977). Handel (1967) believes that the primary issue for a family to solve is the establishment of patterns of separateness and connectedness. Within the family system, one cannot be close to another unless one is a separate entity. Without a clear sense of individual boundaries, family members are fused into an amorphous, undifferentiated ego mass (highly entropic family). Members are not allowed to be individuals or have autonomy. Negentropic families, however, have highly differentiated members with clear self-boundaries. Here, intimacy and individuality can exist together.

Power

This family system variable is concerned with the way power is distributed within the family system. It is made up of two aspects: style and interpersonal power. The style of power in a family system refers to the manner in which a family uses power, that is, is it chaotic, lead by one powerful member, or egalitarian? Families across the continuum use power differently. The entropic family tends to have either a chaotic style of power use or, somewhat better, a rigid and authoritarian style. Negentropic families tend to use an egalitarian style of power (Beavers, 1977).

Individual power, or who holds the power in a family, is a difficult distinction to make. Interpersonal power can be either overt or covert. Overt power is openly acknowledged by the group and is illustrated by observable specifics (e.g., who speaks to whom, who directs activities). Covert power is highly effective but is not group sanctioned. Its nature is illicit, and it is almost impossible to observe until the family directs activity toward family goals. An important thing about covert power is that it can be exerted by individual weakness and helplessness (Beavers, 1977). We have often observed families where an invalid member actually "runs the show."

Family Mythology

All families have a "mythology" or an ongoing shared concept of the qualities and capabilities of family members. Families vary in the degree of congruence between their mythology and reality. Entropic families have an incongruent view of themselves, while negentropic families have a family mythology that closely approximates reality (Beavers, 1977).

Family Goals and Goal-Directed Negotiations

All family systems have overt or covert goals to which they direct their functions. In attainment of goals, families have many problems to solve. Two aspects of problem solving in goal attainment are important: a family's efficiency in arriving at solutions or decisions, and the degree to which a family allows its members to negotiate that solution. At that optimum level of functioning, negentropic families solve problems of goal attainment efficiently and rely on family negotiations to arrive at the decision (Beavers, 1977).

Family Boundaries

Friedman (1981) describes family boundaries as a highly crucial means by which families adapt to outside demands and internal needs. Family boundaries are hypothetically semipermeable and will expand (open) or contract (close), depending upon the amounts of system output or environmental input necessary to meet the family needs. The key to successful family adaptation is said to be selective permeability of the family boundaries. Families can be of two types relative to their boundaries: open and closed. Negentropic families are seen as open, welcoming input from the environment that will initiate system change. Entropic families are, conversely, closed, viewing change as threatening and thus, sealing their boundaries to environmental input.

Family Affect or Feeling

Negentropic families tend to present an enjoyable feeling tone, observable to outsiders. Entropic families, however, present a variety of negative feeling states. Beavers (1977) separates affect into four aspects:

1. *Expressiveness.* Competent families have few proscriptions against members expressing a range of feelings. Disturbed families have many rules against expression of negative feelings, since expression might disrupt tenuous control.
2. *Mood and feeling tone.* This aspect is defined by the perceived feeling an observer receives from a family. Negentropic families vibrate positive feelings; entropic families vibrate negative tones. It is important to remember that a feeling of open anger in a family is far less ominous than either pervasive depression or cynicism, as there still remains some hope for change.
3. *Empathy.* This refers to the capacity of a family member to participate in or vicariously experience another member's feelings, volitions, or ideas. A necessary function of capable families is the ability of members to sense and respond to other members' nonverbal cues. This would be a vital attribute of a family with a newborn infant, who cannot verbally make needs known.
4. *Conflict.* This aspect is ubiquitous in any family. It is indicative of functioning difficulty only if it is chronically unresolved.

Family Intergenerational Patterns/Networks

This variable refers to patterns of interaction a family system, or an individual member, has with members of the extended family. In some theories of family therapy (Boszormenyi-Nagy & Spark, 1973; Speck & Attneave, 1983), family networks are seen as major precipitants of malfunction in the family system, or of symptomology in a family member. Coalitions across generational lines, in a lineal sense (e.g., the grandchild-grandparent subsystem), are seen as potentially problematic for family system integrity. The family and its networks, both lineal and collateral, are seen as the target for intervention and treatment.

Family Roles

Since family subsystems are composed of individuals who occupy certain roles, family theorists have borrowed this variable from small-group theory and made it a crucial component of the family system. Assessment of roles and their function within the family can give great insight into the function of the system (Sedgewick, 1978). A role-function perspective facilitates the observation of the way an individual becomes involved in the family system as a superordinant system of behavior. A role can be seen as a goal-directed pattern or a sequence of acts tailored by the curtural process for transactions a person may carry out in a small group or a given situation (Napier & Whitaker, 1978). Roles can be general, specific, ascribed, or acquired. Several points concerning roles are vital to an understanding of how roles function in family subsystems:

1. All roles are *learned.* A child will learn all social role behavior through imitation, identification, and reciprocal transaction with parents. This learning occurs best within an environment of love and security. Most roles learned in "normal" families are appropriate for the overall social system in question (i.e., they will be "culturally patterned").
2. Roles have *norms* associated with them. Individuals in these roles are expected to follow the norms, with some individual variation.
3. No role exists in isolation; it is always patterned to mesh with a *complementary* or *reciprocal role.*
4. Role occupants have *role expectations* of each other which help determine and orient their responses to each other.
5. Roles are a form of *communication,* which depends on a system of cues, signs, symbols, and meanings shared by the participants. Without communication, meaningful interpretation of each other's role is impossible. Response of the other helps determine further aspects of

one's role, since the other's behavior is interpreted as approval or disapproval of the role behavior.

6. Role expectations may have complementarity, which is chiefly responsible for harmony and stability in interpersonal relationships. Role reciprocity, when complementary, confers spontaneity upon human behavior, since there is no need continually to evaluate role behavior feedback for approval.

7. Role *conflict* can arise when role partners disappoint each other's expectations. Role conflict engenders tension, anxiety, and hostility and can arise from various sources: (a) not knowing the required role behavior, (b) discrepancy regarding the goals of roles, (c) assuming a role where no legitimate right to that role exists, and (d) discrepancy in cultural value orientations of role partners (many roles pertinent in the family system are defined differently in different cultures).

When considering the roles that individuals assume in a family, it is important to remember that these roles are often shared with other systems in society. There is also frequent conflict over the manner in which the family sees a role fulfilled and the manner in which society sees the same role fulfilled.

Communication Patterns

Another important variable to consider in the family system is the communication that occurs between members. Satir (1967) defines communication as the verbal and nonverbal behavior that occurs within a social context. Family communication techniques give indication of inter- and intrasystem functioning. It is believed by some family theorists that an individual's level of interpersonal functioning is, in part, a result of *functional* and *dysfunctional* communication patterns within the family system. To be a competent adult—that is, to survive as "human"—one must communicate clearly, in order to find out about people and socially appropriate ways of interacting.

Functional communications are said to be complete messages with no ambiguity between word denotations and connotations, where sender channels are kept open for feedback from the receiver of the communication. Dysfunctional communications, on the other hand, contain ambiguous word meanings, have messages that are incomplete, and inappropriately use symbols and abstractions, leading the receiver to overgeneralize and make false assumptions.

Satir (1967) indicates that there are actually two levels of communication that occur in interpersonal relations: *denotative* and *metacommunicative*. The denotative level of communication deals with the
literal content—what the words literally say. The metacommunicative
level, in contrast, is a comment on the literal content and the nature of
the relationship between the persons involved in the communication.
It is a "message about a message," including both verbal and nonverbal modes of communication. An important aspect of communication
patterns in the family system is the "fit" between these two levels. In
dysfunctional communications, the literal (denotative) message can indicate one thing, while the metacommunicative level can indicate
something quite different. This type of communication will produce
great confusion for the receiver. Such a poor fit of levels of communication is closely aligned to the concept of the double-level
message, which is a statement that says one thing and actually means
another. In entropic dysfunctional families, such messages eventually
evolve into double-bind situations, a very important concept in family
therapy. Such situations in a family system have the tendency to evolve
highly dysfunctional family members.

Family Cultural Background

A family's cultural orientation has a profound effect on the way a
family system presents itself. In fact, all previous variables discussed
will vary, depending upon the family's culture. While an in-depth
study of this vital aspect of family system is far beyond the scope of this
chapter and book, let us look at *value orientation,* which will serve here as
an example.

Kluckhohn (1968), an anthropologist, has developed a theory concerning how value orientation will be a factor in the pattern a family
system will assume. Values are deeply rooted in an individual or
family, and they are mainly unconscious and totally pervasive. Value
orientation will be transmitted by the family system to its members
and will affect the pattern of behavior manifest by individual family
members. Kluckhohn has made several assumptions about living: (1)
there are a limited number of common human problems that all
societies must solve in order to survive; (2) all societies do *not* solve
these problems in the same manner, and there is much variability in
the range of solutions; and (3) all variants of all solutions are present in
varying degrees in all societies at all times, although each society has a

dominant value orientation profile, which affects the philosophies of life espoused by its members.

These common problems and a brief description of the values associated with their solution follows:

1. Problem: What is the character of innate human nature? Values: It may be evil, good, or both good and evil.
2. What is the relation of humanity to nature? Values: Humanity may be subjugated to nature, live in harmony with nature, or have mastery over nature.
3. What is the temporal (time-related) focus of human life? Values: It may be past, present, or future oriented.
4. What is the modality of human activity? Values: It may be simply being, being-in-becoming, or doing.
5. What is the modality of people's relationship to others (relational focus)? Values: The focus may be lineal, collateral, or individualistic.

These major variables are treated in this chapter and in family systems theory in general as though they are indigenous to the family system. These variables are also major constructs in other approaches to the study of the family. Throughout this book, these variables will be viewed in relation to their importance to the childbearing family *system*. For the sake of clarity, and to help the reader differentiate between a family systems approach and other approaches to the family, some of these other approaches will be briefly described.

OTHER CONCEPTUAL FRAMEWORKS FOR STUDY OF THE FAMILY

The following frameworks have either evolved from or elaborate the notion of the family system. As such, they are briefly mentioned here, so that the reader may be aware of the total scope of frameworks for viewing the family. In particular, the developmental approach discussed by Duvall (1977) is a vital adjunct to the concept of family system, as it specifies that the family system evolves through a variety of developmental phases. Such a view of the family system is necessary in order to consider it during the phase of pregnancy.

Structural-Functional Approach

Actually an elaboration of an aspect of family systems theory, this approach chooses as its primary goal the study of the family's structural and functional dimensions. According to Thibodeau and Hawkins (1982), this approach posits both an internal system for regulating relations within a family and an external system for dealing with the transactions between the family and outside groups or events.

Interactional Approach

The specific focus in this framework is the manner in which family members relate to each other within the family system. Again, the view is narrowed from the entire system to a specific part of the system, in an effort to understand better one component of the total. This approach seeks to interpret family phenomena in terms of the family's internal dynamics (Friedman, 1981). The core phenomena of the framework are the assessment of roles and the communication process. A weakness of this framework or approach is a failure to consider the family in its interactions with its external environment.

Institutional Approach

The family is observed, in this framework, as an institution of society. Core concerns are the family's relation to other institutions in society and to the cultural values of that society. The primary focus, then, is on the function that a family has for society, how these functions compare with functions of other institutions, and how family functions change over time (Friedman, 1981; Thibodeau & Hawkins, 1982).

Developmental Approach

In this framework, the family system is seen as growing and developing over its own life cycle. Like an individual system, a family system passes through predictable, sequential stages from its inception through its dissolution, each stage complete with developmental tasks the family must master (Friedman, 1981; Thibodeau & Hawkins, 1982). As might be expected, pregnancy is one major phase of the family life cycle. Thus, the framework of family system development proposed by Duvall (1977) provides an important indicator of psychosocial dimensions in the family. This aspect of family response to pregnancy will be discussed in the following chapter.

A GLOSSARY OF IMPORTANT SYSTEMS TERMS

Von Bertalanffy, the founder of general systems theory, first defined systems theory in 1945 as the study of the relationship of interactional parts in context (Von Bertalanffy, 1971). He classified systems by the way their components are organized (interrelated) and the identified laws or typical patterns of behavior for the different classes of systems. Miller (1969), another systems theorist, defined systems theory as "A set of related definitions, assumptions, and propositions which deal with reality as an integrated hierarchy of organizations of matter and energy (p. 87)." The evolution of systems theory brought many new concepts to the foreground. Since basic understanding of such concepts is imperative to understanding a system, of which the family is one type, some of the key concepts will be briefly discussed.

System. Kanter and Lehr (1975) define a system as a set of different things or parts that meets two requirements: (1) the parts are directly or indirectly related to one another in a network of reciprocal causal effects and (2) each component part is related to one or more other parts of the set in a stable but dynamic manner at any given time. The system and its environment make up a universe, which is the totality of what should be studied in a given situation (Friedman, 1981).

Open System. All living systems must be open systems. Such a system interacts with its environment, exchanging matter and energy (inputs and outputs). Such environmental interaction is deemed necessary for survival (Friedman, 1981).

Closed System. A closed system is one in which, theoretically, no interchange occurs with the environment. Such a system would be self-contained and not interdependent with the environment. Since no truly closed system has yet been isolated in reality, Parsons and Bales (1955) indicate that a closed system is one in which there is a relative lack of energy exchange across a boundary between the system and the environment.

Boundary. Each system has a boundary or a limiting membrane that differentiates it from its environment. In living systems, the boundary is both limiting and permeable, allowing necessary interaction with the outer world but maintaining system integrity. Boundary permeability is an important characteristic of a system, since the exchange of matter and energy between system and environment affects attainment of system equilibrium (Beavers, 1977).

Negentropy. A state of highly complex order within a system is called negentropy (Beavers, 1977). As a system grows in a positive manner, through its interactions with its environment, it evolves increasingly complex and ordered structures within its boundaries. As it grows, the negentropic system simultaneously evolves power and control over these ordered structures. Such complexity of ordered structures within the system allows for adaptiveness, tolerance to change, flexibility, and increased differentiation of subsystems. Negentropy denotes a high state of evolution for a system.

Entropy. The converse of negentropy, entropy is a term that describes the tendency of things to go into disorder (Georgescu-Roegen, 1971). Entropic systems lose power and control over their chaotic structures and have no flexibility or adaptiveness. This rigid, disordered structure is characteristic of closed and dead systems.

Hierarchy. Systems are arranged in a hierarchy of levels. A system may consist of a number of units of a sort characteristic of one level of organization below the system referred to (Beavers, 1977). Conversely, the same system might contain one or several component units of a system one level of organization above it. For example, one hierarchy of systems, from lowest to highest order, is as follows: cell→tissue →gastrointestinal system→human organism→family→community →cultural group→(and so on). When using a systems framework, it is necessary to identify the target or focal system being assessed. This system, then, represents the whole that is being studied. Lower-level systems become parts (subsystems) of the focal system and are seen only in terms of their interactions within the system. Knowledge of any one part cannot, in itself, give knowledge of the focal system without consideration of the total interaction of all parts in the focal system. That is, knowledge of the gastrointestinal subsystem cannot tell us all we need to know about the human individual without consideration of the individual's total structure and function.

Feedback. Feedback refers to the process by which a system monitors the internal and environmental responses (input) to its behaviors (output) (Friedman, 1981). A further aspect of feedback is the system's response to receipt of input from the environment, through the alteration of its output.

Adaptation. This systems concept depends on the system's maintaining enough stability for coherent identity while making necessary accommodations to its changing world (Beavers, 1977). Adaptation may be seen as a component of feedback (Friedman, 1981), since it indicates system adjustment to input; however, it implies more. It implies the ability of the system to maintain a necessary minimum predictable state (homeostasis/morphogenesis) while changing in response to input and evolving new structures (morphogenesis). There is no static state in living systems; change is a constant state leading to progression or regression. Rigidity of a system, then, impedes its ability to adapt.

Time. Time is an integral part of living systems and is marked by system change through growth, development, aging, and death (Beavers, 1977).

Progressive Differentiation. This term denotes the manner in which systems grow (Beavers, 1977). A living system is capable of progressively advancing to a state of higher complexity and organization through interchange with the environment (state of negentropy). The converse of progressive differentiation, then, might be system regression to a state of disorder or entropy.

Value Hierarchy. Within a system, all needs and responses are not of equal value. Some are considered by the system as more important than others. Choosing the most important need or response is a characteristic of all living systems. Such values may be determined by observing how a system responds to stress. Values become apparent as the system functions to meet the stress and arrive at choices (Beavers, 1977).

Isomorphism. This is the presence of similar structures in seemingly dissimilar systems. One may find similar structure at different levels of a hierarchy (Beavers, 1977). An example might be that the structure observed in a family is a microcosm of the structure of the society.

REFERENCES

Beavers, W. R. (1977). *Psychotherapy and growth: A family systems perspective*. New York: Brunner/Mazel.

Boszormenyi-Nagy, I., & Spark, G. (1973). *Invisible loyalties*. New York: Harper & Row.

Bowen, M. (1978). The use of family theory in clinical practice. In M. Bowen (Ed.), *Family therapy in clinical practice*. New York: Jason Aronson.

Duvall, E. N. (1977). *Marriage & family development*. Philadelphia, PA: Lippincott.

Friedman, M. (1981). *Family nursing*. New York: Appleton-Century-Crofts.

Georgescu-Roegen, N. (1971). *The entropy law and the economic process*. Cambridge, MA: Harvard University Press.

Handel, G. (1967). *The psychosocial interior of the family*. Chicago, IL: Aldine.

Kanter, D., & Lehr, W. (1975). *Inside the family*. New York: Harper & Row.

Kluckhohn F. (1968). Variation in the basic values of family systems. In N. Bell & E. Vogel (Eds.), *A modern introduction to the family*. New York: Free Press.

Miller, J. G. (1969). Living systems: Basic concepts. In W. Gray, F. Buhl, & N. Rizzo (Eds.), *General systems theory and psychiatry*. Boston: Little, Brown.

Napier, A., & Whitaker, C. (1978). *The family crucible*. New York: Harper & Row.

Parsons, T., & Bales, R. (1955). *Family socialization and interaction process*. New York: The Free Press.

Satir, V. (1967). *Conjoint family theory*. Palo Alto, CA: Science and Behavior Books.

Sedgewick, R. (1978). The family as a system: A network of relationships. In B. Backer, P. Dubbert, & E. Eisenman (Eds.), *Psychiatric/mental health nursing: Contemporary readings*. New York: Van Nostrand.

Sherwen, L. (1981). *Introduction to family theory*. Lecture at Rutgers School of Nursing, Newark, NJ, Sept. 21.

Speck, R., & Attneave, C. (1983). *Family networks*. New York: Pantheon Books.

Thibodeau, J., & Hawkins, J. (1982). *Primary care nursing: Crisis model in client management*. Monterey, CA: Wadsworth.

Von Bertalanffy, L. (1971). Systems, symbols and the image of man. In I. Galdston (Ed.), *The interface between psychiatry and anthropology*. New York: Brunner/Mazel.

Chapter 2

The Pregnant Family: Structure and Function

The previous chapter indicated that the family system, as an integrated entity, may grow and develop in a sequential fashion, much in the manner that an individual system develops. The focus of this chapter is on family growth and development through one of the most important phases of the family life cycle—that of childbearing. With the advent of children, a major reorganization of family structure and function will be necessary. Such major reorganization of a system has been seen to produce a crisis state, here seen as a developmental crisis. We will discuss nursing interventions designed to assist the pregnant family in the developmental crisis of reorganization to incorporate a new member.

FAMILY SYSTEM DEVELOPMENT

In 1974, Minuchin described the family developmental cycle as a key component of any schema based on viewing the family as a system. Such a concept originated in the 1950s with Duvall (1977), who saw the family itself as a basic unit of development. The family system, like the individual system, grows and changes and, as a whole, has its own developmental tasks (Carter & McGoldrick, 1980). Such a concept was an inevitable outgrowth of the theories concerned with individual growth and development and of systems theory in general, with its concept of isomorphism. In her book, *Marriage and Family Development,* Duvall (1977) describes certain concepts that are important in understanding how the family system develops. We will discuss some of these in this section.

Family Developmental Tasks

Family developmental tasks are those basic family tasks that are specific to a given stage of development in the family life cycle. They are directed toward maintaining family well-being and continuation at any particular period during that life cycle. Family developmental tasks are seen, by Duvall (1977), as the growth responsibilities a family must accomplish at its particular stage of development (1) to satisfy its biological requirements, (2) to meet its cultural imperatives, and (3) to satisfy its own aspirations and values.

A family, similar to an individual, can achieve success or failure in meeting the tasks or growth responsibilities that arise at various stages in the life cycle. Family success in mastering current tasks leads to success in mastering subsequent tasks that will arise in new developmental phases. Failure, however, will lead to difficulty with later family developmental tasks and to disapproval from society (Duvall, 1977).

Family developmental tasks arise when the needs of one or more family members converge with the expectations of society in terms of family performance. Internal (subsystem) tension and pressure combine with societal expectations (input) to produce a necessity for family system change. The need for change, which can be viewed as a developmental crisis for the family, engenders new tasks that must be mastered by the family in order to resolve the crisis, restore homeostasis, and ready itself for subsequent stages of development.

Duvall and others have identified critical stages where these conditions will exist and the family will need to solve stage-critical developmental tasks. Duvall's focus is primarily on childrearing; thus, critical events marking the stages are family-related phenomena such as getting married, giving birth, launching young adults, and adjusting to the "empty next." Stress on the family system is inevitable during these stages of growth over the life cycle and gives impetus to family solution of developmental tasks. This picture may be complicated, however, by unpredictable events during the life cycle, such as birth of a defective child, untimely death of a member, or natural disasters. Thus, family systems, as well as individual systems, may have situational crises as well as normal, expected developmental crises where family developmental tasks are expected and predictable (Carter & McGoldrick, 1980).

Duvall's Eight-Stage Family Life Cycle

The following lists Duvall's (1977) eight stages of family development and gives the context for understanding the developmental phase of the beginning family. Although other theoreticians have elaborated this schema, it is still the predominant mode of viewing the family life cycle.

Stage 1 Beginning: Married couple without children

Stage 2 Childbearing: Oldest child under 30 months

Stage 3 Preschool: Oldest child 30 months to 6 years

Stage 4 School: Oldest child 6 to 13 years

Stage 5 Teenage: Oldest child 13 to 20 years

Stage 6 Launching: Period between the leaving of the oldest child and the youngest child

Stage 7 Middle: "Empty next" until retirement

Stage 8 Aging: Retirement to death of both spouses

Developmental Tasks for the Early Family

The basic stage-specific family tasks (Duvall, 1977) in the establishment phase of marriage (dependent upon the couple's social status, ethnic and racial group, and family background) are

1. Finding, furnishing, and maintaining a first home
2. Establishing mutually satisfactory means of support
3. Allocating responsibilities
4. Establishing mutually acceptable personal, emotional, and sexual roles
5. Interacting with in-laws, other relatives, and the larger community
6. Planning for possible children (including contraceptive use, decision to have children, and dealing with pregnancy)
7. Maintaining couple motivation and morale

Developmental Tasks of the Childbearing Family

This stage of the family life cycle begins with the birth of the first baby and continues until the firstborn is of preschool age. During this phase, husband and wife must make the difficult transition to being parents, a process that will continue to be a focus in later chapters in this book. This includes:

1. Arranging space (territory) for a child
2. Financing childbearing and childrearing
3. Assuming mutual responsibility for child care and nurturing
4. Facilitating role learning of family members; that is, assuming the maternal and paternal roles
5. Adjusting to changed communication patterns in the family to accommodate a newborn and young child
6. Planning for subsequent children
7. Realigning intergenerational patterns; that is, establishment of grandparent-grandchild subsystems
8. Maintaining family members' motivation and morale
9. Establishing family rituals and routines (Duvall, 1977)

CRISIS AND THE CHILDBEARING FAMILY

The family, in this chapter, has been described as a system that undergoes development, growth, and change. As with individual systems, growth and development through stages of the life cycle produce crises (maturational or developmental) for the family system. A brief review of crisis theory will set the stage for the family developmental crisis of childbearing (pregnancy).

Crisis has commonly been used as a model for intervention in nursing. While it can be used for assessing individual systems, it is also highly useful for analyzing the family system in distress. It is based, in addition, on the developmental stage concept in its incorporation of developmental crisis. The concept of crisis contains both positive and negative aspects. If handled well by the system, it allows for a higher, more complex level of functioning, through incorporation of new coping strategies. If handled poorly by the system, however, crisis can lead to a decline in the level of system function (Thibodeau & Hawkins, 1982).

Parad and Caplan (1969), in their classic work, define crisis as the impact of any event that challenges the assumed state of the world and forces the individual to change his view of, or readapt to, the world, to himself, or both. They indicate that, when a crisis occurs, there is a period of disequilibrium that overpowers the system's homeostatic mechanisms. The system (family or individual) is then faced with problems that are of basic importance, since they are linked with inherent needs. Conversely, these problems cannot be solved quickly by means of the system's normal range of problem-solving mechanisms. Life events likely to induce a crisis have two broad criteria: they are of basic importance to the system and resist solution by familiar methods. Such events, according to Caplan and Parad, include pregnancy, birth, and role transitions. Problems evolved from such events demand solutions from the system that are often novel in light of previous life experience.

Whether the system resolves the crisis in a positive or negative manner is dependent upon a variety of factors (1) the nature of the crisis event, (2) the state of organization or disorganization of the system at the point of impact, (3) the resources of the system, and (4) the system's previous experience with crisis (Le Masters, 1969). Actually, three outcomes are possible for crisis resolution: System homeostasis will be restored at a higher level of functioning, it will remain at the same level as before the crisis, or it will fall to a lower level of functioning.

Thibodeau and Hawkins (1982) indicate that crisis is a self-limited, temporal state. The system cannot remain in a state of disequilibrium for more than six weeks. During this time, the crisis may be successfully resolved or it may be unsuccessfully resolved, leading to major disorganization of the system (entropy).

Parad (1969) indicates that there are two types of crises: maturational or developmental, and situational or accidental. Situational crises are seen as unexpected, stressful external events and may or may not coincide with a developmental crisis. Maturational or developmental crises, which are what concerns us in this chapter, are somewhat different. They are seen as "normal" since most systems experience them routinely in the process of growth and development. They are generally viewed as periods of marked physical, psychological, and social change that are characterized by disturbances in pattern. During these periods, a combination of biopsychosocial stimuli poses certain tasks that must be faced and mastered with a reasonable degree of effectiveness if the next maturational stage is to yield its full potential for further growth and development.

One of the first individuals to postulate parenthood as a crisis was

LeMasters (1969). He reasoned that, since a family is a small social system, the adding of a new member will force a reorganization of the system as dramatic as the removal of a member. While this reorganization and subsequent crisis is most profound for the first child, all subsequent births will produce the necessity to reorganize and hence cause a variant of the first developmental crisis of childbearing. Based on his studies and clinical work, LeMasters makes several conclusions concerning parenthood as a crisis state:

1. Parenthood (and not marriage) is highly romanticized in our culture. Middle-class couples often unexpectedly find their new parental roles to be in conflict with socioeconomic and other roles.
2. Couples are seldom trained for parenthood. There is little available in society to prepare husbands and wives to become fathers and mothers.
3. Birth of an infant forces immediate reorganization of the two-person pattern of group interaction into a triangle pattern. This is painful, especially if one member of the previous pair (often the father) is forced into the position of semi-isolate.
4. Parenthood marks the final transition to maturity and adult responsibility in our society. The couple now has achieved a certain parity with their own parents (LeMasters, 1969). Further, this step marks another phase of separation-individuation from parent.

Since LeMasters developed his theory, several investigators and theoreticians have challenged this notion of pregnancy as a crisis (Grossman, Eichler, & Winickoff, 1980; Leifer, 1980; Wolkind, & Zajicek, 1981). Lederman (1984) indicates that, based on her research it seems more appropriate to "conceptualize the normal course of childbearing as a test which comes as part of growth, and as a challenge rather than a crisis" (p. 13). This view, however, is not at all inconsistent with Parad's (1969) view of a normal developmental crisis discussed earlier in this chapter. Crisis, especially a developmental crisis, is not inherently a positive or negative event. It is a period of great physical, psychological, and social change in which certain tasks must be faced and mastered by the system. The challenge comes in the successful mastering of these developmental tasks, leading the family to a higher level of functioning.

There is another important reason to continue to regard childbearing as a classical developmental crisis, for purposes of this chapter. Crisis theory has been extensively investigated, both theoretically and clinically; hence, there are empirically documented interventions that professionals have developed for use in resolving a crisis and assisting the family to attain a higher level of functioning. Inherent in the concept of crisis is a period of system "openness" to interventions of a professional, actions that will help the system (here, the family) develop a higher-level resolution to the new, changed situation. The concept of a developmental challenge or test does not necessarily carry such a connotation and may in fact imply that the family should pass its childbearing test or challenge alone.

To summarize, childbearing will be viewed as a developmental crisis for the family system. Within the system, a variety of changes in structure, function, and existing subsystems will occur. Pregnancy, and the perinatal period initiate reorganization of the family system; indeed, many of the changes must be completed before the infant is actually on the family scene. The chapters in this book will focus, in depth, on changes that will occur in the family system and its members during pregnancy. The following section will give a brief overview of some of these changes.

OVERVIEW OF THE PREGNANT FAMILY

Many of the important variables within the family will change during pregnancy and the perinatal period. Such necessity to change will produce a developmental (maturational) crisis for the family. The manner in which the pregnant family restructures itself and readjusts its goals and functions is important in the overall movement of the family along the wellness continuum (that is, its movement toward negentropy, rather than entropy).

Structure

Perhaps the most dramatic changes for the family system are alterations in structure. LeMasters (1969) mentions the problems that occur with the addition of a new member, especially with the first pregnancy. The movement from a stable dyadic structure to a volatile triangle with its shifting patterns of interaction is always a stress. Complexification of the triangling network with addition of a fourth or fifth member is also difficult and multiplies the interaction patterns that may occur. All family members must learn, occasionally, to be the "isolate" or the member who is temporarily left out of a communication.

When considering the shift in structure, it is important to remember that the fetus is as much a part of the triangle as the newborn will be.[1] During this fetal phase of the shift from dyad to triangle, the father almost invariably takes the position of isolate. It is difficult for him to relate to and indeed even conceptualize the fetus as human, especially before he can actually feel fetal movement. After the birth, the father has traditionally been the "outsider," with the mother-newborn symbiotic pair being the interacting parts of the triangle. The current emphasis on father "bonding" and involvement in care of the newborn may alter this pattern. Occasionally, then, the mother may find herself the left-out member of the triangle.

In addition to alteration to a triangle form of structure (or a networking of shifting triangles with subsequent pregnancies), the family must establish additional subsystems. The husband-wife subsystem must expand to include a mother-child and father-child subsystem; the firstborn child may later have to learn to function in a sibling subsystem; and so on.

Power

The assessment of the power patterns in a family will become more complex or may change during pregnancy. An egalitarian dyad may slip into more traidtional male-female power positions during pregnancy. The father may make all "instrumental" decisions regarding the pregnancy and literally attempt to "manage" it. This paternal reaction toward pregnancy will be discussed in more depth in Chapter 8.

---

[1]The third "member" of a triangle does not necessarily have to be a real, viable human; in fact it can even be a pet, a dead loved one, an ideal, or an idea. Watzlawick most fascinatingly discusses this point in his classic analysis of the play, "Who's Afraid of Virginia Woolf?" In the play, George and Martha, the main protagonists, maintain a triangle relationship with an imaginary son (Watzlawick, Beavin, & Jackson, 1967).

It was mentioned in the preceding chapter that weakness in an individual can also be a highly powerful tool. Sometimes through sheer helplessness the newborn (or even the fetus) holds much power in a family, dictating many behaviors and activities of the parents.

Boundaries

Pregnancy may necessitate a shift in both subsystems boundaries and in the total family boundary. On a subsystem level, the pregnant woman enters the unique state of containing a "field within a field." Her wholeness incorporates within it another human field or system (fetus) which is not quite separate and not quite part of her own pattern and organization. The mother and fetus are said to be in a state of biological symbiosis, sharing a common "membrane" or boundary. Another alteration the woman may undergo is a desire to make her boundary more protective or impenetrable. The mother-to-be may see her body as a protective container for her fetus and may try to reduce stimuli coming into her system.

The father, on the other hand, is faced with giving support, love, and his own energy to his wife, who is closing in on herself and becoming more and more internalized. In order to give input to his wife, his boundaries must be highly permeable and in effect he must expand to experience an empathy with her, even while his wife's boundaries are closing in around her. Such a paradox in subsystem interactions can require intervention from health care professionals and will be discussed in Chapter 7.

On the family system level, the family boundary must become highly permeable to selected input. The family must receive much care and educational input from many environmental sources if it is to cope successfully with both the physical and psychological aspects of pregnancy.

Affect or Feeling Tone

Alteration in family feeling tone during pregnancy may signal an unresolved conflict in the process of reorganization. The nurse, when perceiving a chronic negative feeling tone, would need to observe or question further to determine the source of the unresolved problem in the family system. For example, variations in cultural beliefs concerning roles discussed in the next section may produce great conflict and attending negative feeling tone in the pregnant family.

Family Interactional Patterns

Interactional patterns include both role interactions and communication patterns, both of which must change during pregnancy and the perinatal period. The changes associated with parental role assumption will be dramatic during the first pregnancy and will receive much attention in Chapter 5. Both the woman and man must go through this process before the infant actually arrives. Aspects of role assumption, such as fantasy production (Chapters, 5, 6, & 8), will also receive attention. In addition, it is at this point that cultural variations in parental roles may produce great conflict. Each culture has a well-ingrained concept of how "mother" or "father" should behave. It will be easy to disappoint a partner's cultural expectations of one's role behavior if one does not come from the same cultural background.

Communication patterns will change in the pregnant family, according to the changed structure (triangle or triangling network). Members of the triangle will need to learn to take turns communicating, since only two members can communicate at any one time. When individuals have been communicating as a two-person structure, communicating in a triangle structure can produce stress and tension in the system.

The Family System and Its Environment

As a system that is rearing and socializing children, the family will receive input from many other systems in its environment. Since the family has a mandate to develop individuals who will fit into society, a given culture, and a given extended family, many institutions and systems have a stake in how the family rears its children. Societal expectations of parental roles and functions may be in conflict with family expectations. Input from the environment can also produce stress and tension for the childbearing family system.

NURSING INTERVENTION FOR THE PREGNANT FAMILY

It has been the thesis of this chapter that pregnancy and childbearing require great change in the structure of a family. Such change and its accompanying stress produces a developmental crisis for the family. The crisis of childbearing produces developmental tasks for the family to master to attain a higher level of growth and complexity (negentropy). Evolution of new coping strategies is necessary for the family to master its tasks and move along to a higher level of function. It is not surprising, then, that a model for nursing intervention with the pregnant family comes from crisis theory.

Thibodeau and Hawkins (1982) provide an excellent framework for working with an individual in crisis. It may be simply adapted to accommodate the pregnant family in the developmental crisis of childbearing. The goal of nursing intervention, according to Thibodeau and Hawkins, is to assist the client (here, the pregnant family) to capitalize on the growth potential inherent in the crisis. Interventions occur at three levels: the precrisis state, the crisis state, and the postcrisis state.

Precrisis is described as a state of dynamic equilibrium where the system is in harmony with the environment. Depending on the developmental state of the family, this system will be subject to predictable risks (developmental events) in the course of the life cycle. The family that intends to move into the phase of childbearing will undergo predictable changes. Thus, the nurse will be able to intervene at a primary health care level—the level designed to prevent problems and promote strengths. By intervening with anticipatory guidance for the childbearing family, the nature of the crisis event associated with the addition of a new member may be ameliorated. This, in turn, will facilitate crisis resolution, mastering of developmental tasks, adaptation to restructuring and movement to a higher, more complex level of functioning.

In addition to anticipatory guidance, Thibodeau and Hawkins (1982) also suggest that the nurse provide the following, during the precrisis phase, for the client (pregnant family system): (1) assessment of risk factors to detect potential areas of weakness; (2) assessment of strengths as well as weaknesses; (3) assessment of past coping and problem-solving strategies; (4) appropriate screening procedures; (5) identification of resources (inside and outside the system); (6) health teaching; and (7) assistance with health promotion or maintenance strategies. In addition, it would be vital to assess the family's past history in dealing with crisis.

Crisis will occur in a system when the current repertoire of responses and coping strategies is no longer sufficient to deal with the newly evolved problems posed by development. While Thibodeau and Hawkins (1982) maintain that all crises, including developmental crises, can be avoided, this book will take the view that the crises of development are inevitable. A system must learn new behaviors, responses, and coping strategies to deal with new, higher-level tasks evolved in a new developmental phase. Nothing in the previous level of development prepares a system to deal with all new tasks. Thus, some degree of crisis and system disorganization is necessary to allow new responses to emerge. The severity of the crisis and whether these new behaviors and responses move the system toward negentropic (higher-level) functioning is dependent upon the level of nursing intervention in the precrisis and crisis phases.

Thibodeau and Hawkins (1982) indicate that the specific aim of crisis intervention is to restore the indivdiual to the precrisis level of functioning. This may be amended according to the model of family system growth and wellness, wherein the aim is to facilitate system movement to a level higher than precrisis functioning (negentropy). The nurse interacts with the system in order to reduce the impact of the event (here, childbearing) and to capitalize on system strengths.

Rapoport (1969) identifies three parts to the process of intervention in a crisis; (1) clarification of the problem, (2) acceptance of the client (family) in their current emotional state, and (3) use of appropriate interpersonal and institutional resources in crisis resolution.

Aquilera (1982) poses four steps in crisis intervention:

1. *Assessment.* The problem and its ramifications should be analyzed.
2. *Planning of intervention.* A plan of intervention should be devised to restore the system to at least a precrisis level of functioning. Especially with a pregnant family, the care plan should include moving the system to a higher level of functioning.
3. *Active intervention.* The system (family) should be assisted in (a) gaining understanding of the crisis; (b) expressing feelings openly, (c) exploring alternative means of problem solving. In a developmental crisis, this might require evolving new means of problem solving; and (d) using new resources and strategies.
4. *Resolution of crisis and future planning.* Reinforcement should be given for system (family) behaviors, responses, and strategies that

are successful (here, in meeting and mastering developmental tasks). The system (family) should be helped in planning for the future.

Thibodeau and Hawkins (1982) include a postcrisis phase as a period for nursing intervention. At this point, the time-limited crisis has been resolved by the system, either leading to a higher, the same, or lower level of function. Thibodeau and Hawkins advocate the following nursing interventions during the postcrisis period; (1) measures to support the system in its new strategies of resolution; (2) measures to emphasize inherent growth potential; and (3) measures to reverse or lessen effects of maladaptation to the crisis through appropriate rehabilitative effort or therapy.

The foregoing nursing interventions for the family system in crisis are, necessarily, broad and general. The nurse needs to assess each pregnant family and adapt such interventions to the family system's unique needs and attributes. The following chapters will give more insight into specific forms of intervention, dependent on unique aspects of the pregnant family system.

REFERENCES

Aquilera, D. (1982). *Crisis intervention: Theory and methodology.* St. Louis: C. V. Mosby.

Carter, E., & McGoldrick, M. (1980). The family life cycle and family therapy: An overview. In E. Carter & M. McGoldrick (Eds.), *The family life cycle.* New York: Gardner Press.

Duvall, E.N. (1977). *Marriage and family development* (5th ed.). Philadelphia: Lippincott.

Grossman, F. K., Eichler, L. S., & Winickoff, S. A. (1980). *Pregnancy, birth and parenthood.* San Francisco: Jossey-Bass.

Lederman, R. P. (1984). *Psychosocial adaptation in pregnancy.* Englewood Cliffs, NJ: Prentice-Hall.

Leifer, H. (1980). *Psychological effects of motherhood: A study of first pregnancy.* New York: Praeger.

LeMasters, B. E. (1969). Parenthood as crisis. In H. Parad (Ed.), *Crisis intervention: Selected readings.* New York: Family Service Association of America.

Minuchin, S. (1974). *Families and family therapy.* Cambridge, MA: Harvard University Press.

Parad, H. (1969). Introduction to part II. In H. Parad (Ed.), *Crisis intervention: Selected readings.* New York: Family Services Association of America.

Parad, H., & Caplan, S. (1969). A framework for studying families in crisis. In H. Parad, (Ed.), *Crisis intervention: Selected readings.* New York: Family Services Association of America.

Rapoport, L. (1969). The state of crisis; some theoretical considerations. In H. Parad (Ed.), *Crisis intervention: Selected readings.* New York: Family Services Association of America.

Thibodeau, J., & Hawkins, J. (1982). *Primary care nursing: Crisis model in client management.* Monterey, CA: Wadsworth Health Science Division.

Watzlawick, P., Beavin, J., & Jackson, D. (1967). *Pragmatics of human communication.* New York: W. W. Norton.

Wolkind, S., & Zajicek, E. (1981). *Pregnancy: A psychological and social study.* New York: Grune & Stratton.

Chapter 3

Assessing the Pregnant Family

Cynthia B. Hughes

This chapter will focus on presenting a framework for assessing the childbearing family system. The framework is drawn from systems theory, which defines the family as hierarchical in nature and comprised of units of interacting parts. The childbearing family, like other family units, is comprised of individual subsystems, and the dyads of husband-wife, mother-fetus (child,), father-fetus (child), and sibling-fetus (sibling). The family as a system and its interacting levels form a structure through which assessment of the childbearing family takes place (see Figure 3-1).

Another part of the supporting framework for assessment derives from the family systems theory literature. Key concepts that are meaningful for the pregnant family include *differentiation, distancing-closeness, multigenerational transmission, family emotional system, sibling position, and triangles* (Bowen, 1978). Each one of these family system concepts has relevance at all subsystem levels (see Figure 3-1). In other words, the process of differentiation occurs as a task at the individual level, at the dyad level, and at the family system level. At the family system level family differentiates itself within the community in relation to other families. It also aims to accomplish the task of fostering differentiation of its individual subsystems by promoting an environment in which true self can flourish. (Although we will discuss these concepts, the reader may refer to Chapter 1 for more in-depth definitions.)

The childbearing family will be examined from a systems approach using these specific family concepts. Key assesment features of each subsystem level will be highlighted as they particularly relate to the childbearing family. Specific assessment techniques will be identified.

FAMILY SYSTEM ASSESSMENT CONCEPTS DEFINED

Differentiation Profiles

A key task of families is to produce well-organized and well-integrated individuals with a strong sense of self. Assessing families for this characteristic, for a level of well-defined self versus a so-called pseudo-self[1] gives clues to family health. The emphasis is on whether intellectual skills are used to solve problems and make decisions, or if an individual perspective can be maintained in family situations where emotional involvement is high. The activity level of individuals is assessed to provide further information on individual differentiation. Are individual family members primarily investing their time in maintaining emotional relationships, or is their activity goal directed, toward, for example, childrearing, vocational pursuits, or community involvement? Bowen (1978) correlated low levels of physical as well as psychological health with low levels of differentiation. Collecting data on the physical and mental status of individuals will contribute to the information on levels of differentiation. (See Table 3–4 later in this chapter.)

Distancing-Closeness Dichotomy

Bowen (1978) identifies the basic emotional dilemma facing an individual as togetherness versus separateness. Families are assessed for

---

[1]The pseudo-self is contrasted with the solid-self, which is made up of clearly defined beliefs, opinions, convictions and life principles which are internally consistent and stable, even in situations of high anxiety and stress. The pseudo-self is acquired under emotional pressure in a relationship: the principles and beliefs underlying the pseudo-self system tend to be inconsistent and change with emotional shifts in the relationship system. (Miller & Winstead-Fry, 1982; Bowen, 1978).

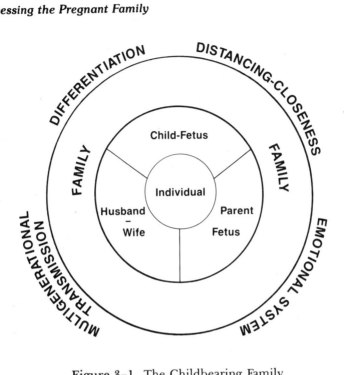

Figure 3-1. The Childbearing Family

this ability to provide both closeness and space. Space is both physical and psychological. When family members have not achieved a balanced sense of closeness or distance, exaggerated behaviors of separation or fusion may occur, such as leaving home to live far away or not being able to leave home at all (i.e., showing severe anxiety such as in school phobia). See Table 3-1 for examples of interview questions addressing this concept.

Multigenerational Transmission Process

Bowen (1978) believes that in order to explain or understand family patterns it is necessary to have information about families for at least three generations. Ways of relating, role evolution, and "scripts" are

Table 3-1. Sample Interview Questions Addressing
Distancing and Closeness

Begin with questions about the physical description of the family residence. Ask about the number of rooms, number of bedrooms, any sharing of bedrooms, places where family members gather together, place where individual family member goes for privacy, etc. Then ask the following.

Who lives at home?
Who lives away from home? Where?
Are there some activities, hobbies, or interests that your family likes to share or to do together. Describe (e.g., ski, go to museums).
Do you or other family members have special activities that interest only you (them)? Are you (they) able to find time for them?
When you have a problem, with whom would you discuss it?
Who do you feel closest to in the family?
Who do you feel most distant from?
How often do you or other family members get off alone?

---

transmitted from generation to generation. People with similar or compatible levels of differentiation and needs marry one another and recreate patterns of interacting or relating that they experience in another generation. Diagraming family members in a "genogram" format can help identify overt patterns as well as covert patterns that are being transmitted from generation to generation (see Figure 3-2). A genogram is a structural framework that enables a nurse quickly and easily to diagram general information (names, occupations, dates of birth, and deaths) as well as more complex information (patterns of overcloseness or conflictual relationships). Certain multigenerational diseases or scripts such as alcoholism or divorce can be easily portrayed (Pendagast, 1978).

Sibling Position

Sibling position is a key concept in understanding families, as certain normative behaviors are associated with certain sibling positions. Acquiring information about each person's sibling position, including the sibling position of adult family members, can provide some broad predictions of behaviors.

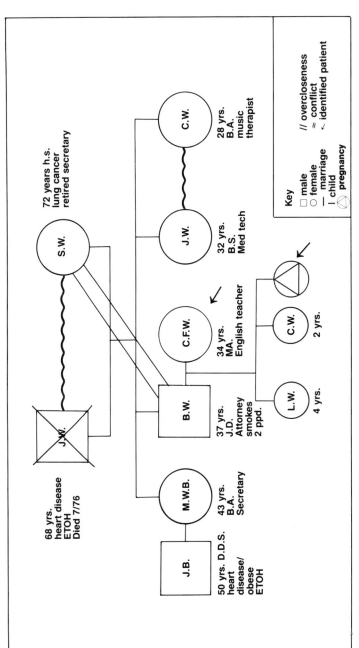

Figure 3-2. Sample Genogram

Triangling

According to Bowen (1978), a two-person interactional subsystem is unstable in a stressful system. To help alleviate the stress or anxiety that builds up in a two-person subsystem, a third person or issue is brought into it. Miller and Winstead-Fry (1982) highlight the automatic and repetitive nature of the less adaptive triangling process. They describe triangles as universal aspects of family life that are actually or potentially present in all families. Families can be assessed for recurring and rigid triangles that occur in their family system, such as two spouses who involve a child in their relationship in place of communicating adult needs and concerns to each other. Fusion or distancing may result from rigid traingles. Table 3-2 provides examples of interview questions that may be used to obtain information related to triangling in families.

Family Emotional System

According to Bowen (1978), the nuclear family emotional system describes the pattern of emotional functioning in a family in a single generation. According to Miller and Winstead-Fry (1982), the emotional system is the force that motivates the family system; the relationship system is the way in which it is expressed in families. Ideally each family has a range of emotional expressions (happiness, sadness, anger) that are available to all family members, and each family member can express his or her own feelings.

Emotional fusion is an outcome of relationships, particularly when individuals are functioning more on an emotional level and less on an

Table 3-2. Sample Interview Questions for Identifying Triangling

Who are you closest to in the family? Most distant from?

Do you have conflicts with one or two people more frequently than others (e.g., mother-in-law, oldest daughter)?

What are these conflicts about? How do they usually end?

How have family members reacted to your pregnancy?

How do your other children (if any) feel about the expected baby? Have they changed their behavior toward you or your spouse in any way?

How does your spouse feel about the expected baby?

Table 3-3. Sample Interview Questions for Evaluating
the Family Emotional System

When you are angry at your spouse, how do you express it? What happens
when you two disagree about something?

Do you find in your family that, if you are angry at a child, your husband will
also feel angry at the child?

If Suzy decided to go on to nursing school instead of law school, how do you
think family members would feel? How would they behave?

When you are angry at your child, how do you express it? When your child is
"naughty," how do you handle the situation?

How do family members express good feelings toward each other?

intellectual level. Fusion is a "togetherness force," a blending of one
person into another. It is contrasted with differentiation, a separateness force, the defining of self. In a fusion situation separate individual
emotions will not be able to be expressed. See Table 3-3 for examples
of interview questions to use in this area.

INDIVIDUAL SUBSYSTEM

The individual as a subsystem in the childbearing family, be she or
he adult or child, woman or man, can be looked at as an individual
with a degree of differenitation having psychological and sociological
characteristics that affect the childbearing phase of family life (see
Table 3-4). For assessment purposes, the psychological aspects can be
further divided into cognitive, emotional, and motivational dimensions, as shown in the table.

Although the physiological dimension is an important indication of
wellness and is related to wellness in the psychological and sociological
realms, the detailed assessment of the physiological status of the pregnant individual is beyond the scope of this book. It is important to interpret physiological signs and symptoms in the context of the
whole individual.

Cognitive assessment of the individual as depicted in Table 3-4
would include such variables as level of education, level of knowledge
of pregnancy and parenting, as well as the general dimensions of
cognitive functioning such as reasoning ability, attention span, and

Table 3-4. Individual (Male or Female) Subsystem
Assessment Areas

Psychological Perspective:

Cognitive Aspects	Affective Aspects	Motivational Aspects
Self-concept	Mood	Interest-involvement
Body image	Intensity	Dependence/independence
Fantasy life	Anxiety/relaxation	Motivation for pregnancy
Education	Dreams	
Knowledge level	Defense mechanisms	
Memory	Emotional range	
Orientation	Emotional stability	
Judgment		
Attention span		
Coping behaviors		
Reasoning/problem solving		

Sociological Perspective:

Age
Socioeconomic status
Role statuses & satisfaction/conflicts with roles
Support systems, for each role
Mothering/fathering relationship history
Sibling order position
Occupational identity; community identity; gender identity

judgment and memory. The client's general knowledge fund about birth and parenting as well as her ability to learn has frequently been related to such variables as seeking early prenatal care, compliance with the therapeutic regime, and pregnancy outcome.

The basic cognitive skills and level of emotional differentiation of an individual are important to an individual's ability to master the developmental tasks that arise during pregnancy. Caplan (1960) states that two important psychological tasks must occur in the childbearing phase: acceptance of the pregnancy and perception of the fetus as a separate individual.

Rubin (1975) discusses four general tasks of the pregnant women: (1) seeking safe passage for herself and her child through pregnancy, labor, and delivery; (2) insuring acceptance of the child she bears by significant persons in her family; (3) binding in to her unborn child; and (4) learning to give of herself. Rubin (1967) has also identified five operations involved in the process of maternal role taking: mimicry, role play, fantasy, introjection-projection-rejection (IPR), and grief work. The operations of mimicry, role play, IPR, and fantasy require the individual to integrate her memories of past pregnant women and mothers with new behaviors and roles she observes in her environment. These behaviors all require functioning cognitive processes. Grief work involves the cognitive dimension in that an individual anticipates, recalls, and reviews those aspects of her current role and lifestyles that may conflict with her new role. Emotionally, a pregnant woman may experience sadness, ambivalence, and anxiety. The healthy balancing of the cognitive and emotional systems is crucial to healthy pregnancy outcome.

Similarities exist between Caplan's and Rubin's views, and these have implications for a well-differentiated individual. Positive acceptance and expression of the pregnancy reflects mastery of intellectual problem-solving skills over the emotional ambivalence and anxiety common in pregnancy. Persistence of ambivalence and lack of acceptance into the second trimester would indicate the lack of resolution of emotional issues as well as a deficit in the cognitive system.

Intrinsic to the outward acceptance of pregnancy are several sociological variables that influence the individual and contribute to a sense of differentiation. An image and concept of mothering and fathering begins with an individual's experience of mothering and fathering in her or his own family of origin. This multigenerational transmission process shapes and directs the newly evolving parenting role in the pregnant family. A woman who has achieved separation and differentiation from her family and holds a positive image and awareness of her own relationship to her parents would have resources that would help her resolve her realistic anxieties and affect her readiness and acceptance of pregnancy. The same is true for a man. Furthermore, achieving a level of differentiation requires an individual to progress through certain developmental tasks, as postulated by a developmental theorist such as Erikson (1963). Since two primary developmental tasks prior to generativity are achieving intimacy and a sense of identity, certain of these characteristics can be evaluated. (Intimacy will be discussed later in the chapter).

Achievement of developmental tasks under most frameworks is

related to age. Pregnancy at a very young age in and of itself would represent a superimposition of additional developmental tasks onto the normal adolescent developmental tasks. Choice of and development of gender, work, and community or occupational roles reflect a development of identity. As an example of the influence of this identity state, Jiminez and Newton (1982) report on a study relating to job orientation and adjustment to pregnancy and early motherhood. Contrary to other studies and reports focusing on role conflict and difficult adjustment to motherhood, they report that women who score high in job commitment have more favorable psychological and emotional experiences in the first pregnancy and postpartum period. Furthermore, the degree of job commitment was not related to maternal attachment behavior. The implication here is that achievement of satisfaction in the work area and all that it entails (occupational identity, sense of positive image, feedback, and work support system) aids in the mothering process.

Changes in the individual emotional system in a childbearing family have also been well documented. The initial response to pregnancy— that of ambivalence—reflects the contradictory emotional states that are evident throughout pregnancy (e.g., joy/sorrow; anticipation/fear). Although lability of mood in the pregnant woman has been physiologically linked to hormonal changes, it contributes to the visibility of the emotional system during pregnancy and can affect the intellectual problem-solving skills of the pregnant individual or the family. As Brazelton (1973) has noted, based on psychoanalytic interviews,

> "The prenatal interviews with normal primiparas . . . uncovered anxiety that often seemed to be of pathological proportions. The unconscious material was so loaded and distorted so near the surface that before delivery one felt an ominous direction for making a prediction about the women's capacity to adjust to the role of mothering. . . . I began to feel that much of the prenatal anxiety and distortion of fantasy could be a healthy mechanism for bringing her out of the old homeostasis" (p. 42).

Other researchers (Caplan, 1960; Rubin, 1972; Sherwen, 1981) have validated these anxious and troubling dreams and fantasies during the childbearing phase, as well as their appearance in a normal population. The nursing assessment of the emotional system in an individual would be based on an awareness of these normal changes occurring during pregnancy. The pregnant individual, although exhibiting an increased intensity and lability of emotions, should still exhibit a normal emotional range and enough stability so that the family may accomplish the tasks of pregnancy.

One of the tenets of the differentiation concept is that people of similar differentiation profiles are attracted to one another (Satir, 1967). Theoretically, then, knowing something about the woman's sense of self or her ability to tolerate closeness will give the nurse information about the pregnant father. For a careful, complete picture of the family and its members, the following assessment factors will be particularly important for the male and his family of origin: past history or perception of fathering and mothering roles, individual psychological status exam, current social network system and its inclusion of fathering figures, perceived awareness of role changes congruent with the paternal role and evidence of acceptance of the pregnancy.

DYADIC SUBSYSTEMS

Husband-Wife

Previous discussion in this chapter has indicated that an important assessment factor in the pregnant family relates to the degree of closeness or distance between the marital pair. The nature of the husband-wife dyad also relates to the sense of differentiation or "I"-ness achieved from their family of origin, where patterns of relating to men and women as spouses were also learned. The multigenerational transmission process is important here, as these are processes directly influenced by an individual's experience with their parents. Assessing these gender roles and intimacy patterns in a previous generation may be helpful to understanding the current family.

The ability to achieve a satisfactory relationship with a partner over time is also important. Several researchers (Hobbs & Cole, 1976;

Table 3-5. Adult Dyad Assessment Areas

Communications:
  Verbal & nonverbal congruence
  Openness
  Quality
  Affect (humor, anger, love, affection)
  Lines of communication (reciprocal, egalitarian, authoritarian)
Perceptions of closeness to or distance from partner
Emotional system:
  Range (ability to express many emotions to each other)
  Depth (intensity, intimacy)
  Stability of emotional/intellectual balance
Sexual components (quality, mutual satisfaction)
Problem solving and task accomplishment (household and financial management, childrearing)
Ability to play (humor, fun, recreation)
Mutually shared goals (parenting and civic responsibilities, values)
Space for individual differences (individual hobbies, interests, sports, friends)

Russell, 1974; Wandersman, Wandersman, & Kahn, 1980) have found associations between the quality of intimacy in the marriage relationship and the ease or difficulty experienced by couples in their transition to parenthood. Broom (1984) points out the customary lack of routine assessment of this aspect of family life during the prenatal or postpartal period.

The nurse can assess the degree of marital intimacy by collecting information on the openness and quality of communication, the partners' perceptions of closeness, the range and depth of emotions partners can share with each other, the satisfaction with the sexual relationship, the ability of the partners to play together as well as manage the problem solving and the work of sharing a home, and, finally, the degree of mutuality of shared goals. These areas of assessment are shown in Table 3-5.

Some changes in the husband-wife relationship result from the pregnancy. Marquart (1976), in a small study of married fathers (N = 15), report that husbands do not see their wives' independence altered. They report an increased protectiveness toward their wives and the unborn child. This was manifested in different ways, such as the father's increased concern for his wife's health or concern for her diet. Marquart (1976) also reported a change in temporal relationships, where men perceived their wives as wanting things done immediately.The nature of the sexual relationship also frequently changes. Husbands and wives have been reported to show both decreased and increased interest in sex. Getting information about the sexual relationship prior to the pregnancy as well as how it has changed and how the partners feel about the change are all important aspects of assessment.

The husbands in Marquart's (1976) study found that the theme of communication changed in the home to focus predominantly on the pregnancy. Husbands also found their social relationships were changed by their seeking out expectant couples or parents of young children more frequently. It is clear that a successful and stable relationship with the father of the child or an adult substitute is important to the health of the pregnancy, but the number of positive and negative extrafamilial systems that have responded to the pregnancy is also important. As Rubin (1975) reports, the woman often assumes the task of influencing the acceptance of pregnancy in those significant others. Based on reciprocal interactional theory, her positive perspective will have an influence on others.

Finally, the fetus may become a third point of a triangle in family relationships. In particular, the fetus intrudes upon the husband-wife relationship. Father may feel the outsider and feel tense and anxious as a result.

Parental-Fetal Subsystem

The sense of self, developed from the family of origin, that the pregnant parent brings to the pregnancy is very important to one of the later tasks of pregnancy, often temporally associated with quickening (about the fifth month of pregnancy). This is the need to attach self to and differentiate self from the developing fetus.

Maternal-fetal interaction has been described as symbiotic, and the term *fusion* has been applied well into the newborn period by some authors but differentiation as a process and task has been identified as beginning as early as the quickening period. Attachment is a parallel process to separation. The parent's ability to perceive the fetus as an individual is integral to the differentiation process. At the same time, attachment, the closeness bonds felt with the developing fetus, is also a significant positive process of pregnancy.

The mother's and father's awareness of the fetus as an individual and separate force with a life and a will of its own, as well their feelings of closeness to it, come most clearly with the parent's perception of its activity and mobility in the uterus and the visibility of unique fetal parts (extremities, head, butt). These things increase the complexity and differentiation of parental imagery and fantasy the parent has about the fetus. This differentiation of the fetus can lead to labeling in the area of temperment—(i.e., peaceful, active) or gender. This differentiation of the fetus as an individual clearly should be positive, congruent with the desired "ideal" baby, and not a fixed or rigid image. A family that exclusively imagines a girl fetus would not be expressing a sense of the separateness of the fetus, but simply a projection of their own desires. Later in pregnancy the mother's willingness to give up the fetus as a separate being is the outcome of the earlier processes of differentiation and attachment. The areas for assessment of this process are shown in Table 3–6.

The maternal-fetal attachment process is clearly related initially to whether or not the pregnancy was planned. A desire for the pregnancy facilitates the positive symbiosis between mother and fetus. Evidence of a mother's positive perception of a changing body image throughout the pregnancy indicates a positive view of the pregnancy. Acknowledging this change by dressing in attractive, appropriate clothes contributes to assessment data of the attachment process.

Pregnant women have anxiety fantasies and dreams related to the fetus but also build up an image of the developing fetus, its position in utero, its development, and its gender. This image can be positive or alien and contributes to the nurses' understanding of the attachment-differentiation process.

Maternal-fetal attachment is observed and identified through body language by the classic portrayal of the mother with her arms hugging her abdomen. Patting the abdomen and singing and talking to the fetus are also documented as signs of mother-fetus attachment. Body language, interaction with the fetus, and imagery of the fetus may all be expected to evolve and in some situations increase in complexity as the pregnancy progresses.

Table 3-6. Areas for Assessment of Maternal-Fetal Attachment and Differentiation

Attachment:
  Planned pregnancy
  Perceptions of changing body image as reflected in grooming, dress
  Fantasy, imagery (normally positive)
  Body language (holding stomach, patting)
  Maternal-fetal interaction (talking, singing)
  Language (use of "we")
  Nesting behaviors (cleaning house, preparing room)
  Protective and health-promoting behaviors (hygiene, nutrition,
    exercise, rest)

Differentiation (through communication, imagery, etc):
  Gender (he, she)
  Fetal position and parts (awareness of head, hands, feet)
  Activity/temperament (quiet, sleepy, active)
  Name (actual or pet name)

The parent who is attached to the fetus would also exhibit protective and health promoting behaviors that would contribute to the well-being of the fetus. Examples of these are eating well, exercising and resting appropriately, and seeking regular health care. Throughout the pregnancy, but especially late in the pregnancy, the parents' attachment and expectations of a unique individual infant would be reflected in nesting behaviors—preparations of the room, house, and layette for the new baby.

Part of nesting or preparation for the new baby is acquiring knowledge about the childbearing and childrearing processes through reading, attending prenatal education classes, or learning new skills, such as care of the infant. Assessment of these behaviors will give clues to the maternal-fetal subsystem.

Recently, more interest has developed in the father's attachment process to the fetus and his involvement with the pregnant state. Herzog (1982), through retrospective interviews, in a sample of fathers experiencing an interruption in the normal pregnancy, has identified certain stages through which the pregnant father may progress. Included in these phases are initially a positive perception of the pregnancy, an enhanced sense of manliness and interest in sexual relations, a turning toward the fatherliness role, and nesting preparations for a big and magical event later in the pregnancy.

In particular, the fathers' complaints of physiological disturbance or pregnancy symptoms (couvade experience) has received attention in the literature. The manifestation of such symptoms has been linked to a close identification and involvement with the pregnancy in certain fathers (those with less education and those with less fathering experience). Antle (1975) suggests that such couvade symptoms may be a "self-acceptable unconscious expression" of the expectant father's pregnant emotional state, in those individuals who do not need to strongly suppress their feminine traits and are not prepared to verbalize their feelings freely (p. 115). The most frequently occurring male pregnancy symptoms reported in the literature are abdominal—nausea, vomiting, and abdominal pain—but other complaints such as sties, backaches, oral cravings, and skin lesions have been linked to this condition. Toothaches have also been reported in an increased rate among pregnant fathers (Hott, 1976, Trethowan & Conlon, 1965).

Besides physical symptoms, 40% of a sample of men in a study by Trethowan and Conlon (1965) reported being anxious, while 21% reported psychiatric symptoms such as depression, tension, insomnia, irritability, nervousness, weakness, headaches, and stuttering. Pregnancy in one sample (Hartman & Nicolay, 1966) has been related to certain acting-out sexual behaviors such as exhibitionism, rape, and homosexual acts in heretofore heterosexual men.

Leonard (1976) interviewed 52 fathers soon after delivery and found that the positive feelings and attitudes fathers exhibited toward their newborns were significantly related to (1) expressed enjoyment in taking care of young children, (2) number of children desired prior to marriage, (3) experience with children, (4) planning of pregnancy, (5) number of children currently desired, and (6) knowledge of baby care.

Fatherliness is a developmental process whereby attachment and differentiation with the fetus evolve throughout the pregnancy. The initial response to news of the expected pregnancy—that of ambivalence—has been reported in fathers (Obzrut, 1976) similar to the ambivalence reported by mothers. Accomplishment of the task of accepting the pregnancy is replaced with a growing awareness of the fetus as a developing individual, concurrent with the development of a fatherly role. The father's involvement with the fetus can be evaluated by behaviors such as accompaniment and involvement in prenatal educational classes, visits to the physician, ability and willingness to assume certain tasks the pregnant mother is temporarily unable to perform, such as lifting. Behaviors such as patting the abdomen and fantasies related to the fetus, also indicate a beginning attachment to the fetus as an individual and the trying on of the role of father.

Reiber (1976) points out the social and cultural nature of the fathering role. A pregnant father who exhibits the traditional masculine roles of task management, toughness, aggressiveness, and competitiveness in his individual and husband styles may carry these over to the fathering role at the expense of the feminine characteristics of nurturing and tenderness. The roles fathers take on during the pregnancy can vary. May (1982) reported that 9 out of 20 fathers reported feeling a little detached or being more of an observer of the pregnancy. This stance of emotional distance was reported in men who also were pleased to be expecting a baby, wanted to be the best possible fathers and were interested in supporting their wives. Many of these men reported a personality style in other situations congruent with this response to pregnancy. Among the roles often emphasized by fathers during pregnancy can be that of the task-manager. This is close to a traditional instrumental portrait of the father who makes decisions, manages finances, solves problems and accomplishes the physical tasks of getting ready for the new baby.

Assessing the role taken on by the father is important in describing the nature of the role and the congruence with the mother's expectations and needs. Areas for assessment are shown in Table 3–7. (See also Table 3–4.)

Table 3–7. Paternal-Fetal Assessment Areas

Planned pregnancy
Perception of pregnancy (positive, negative)
Couvade experience (nausea and vomiting, fatigue, weight change)
Past experience with children
Past experience of father role
Pregnant fathering role (task-manager, observer)
Nesting behavior (preparing room, planning finances)
Differentiation of fetus (gender, name, temperament, activity)
Body language directed toward fetus (patting, feeling abdomen, protective behavior toward mother, hugging wife)

Sibling-Fetal Dyad

Little is written in the literature related to the sibling's attachment to the fetus and the sibling's growing awareness of the fetus as a separate child. The child's behavior and understanding of the pregnancy will be related to the child's emotional and cognitive development. What will become evident is the triangular nature of the relationship between the child and the fetus. Since the young child is still very oriented toward the parents, the perception of the fetus will be related to the parent-child relationship and the fulfillment of the child's individual needs. A child frequently will picture the fetus in her or his own image and request a sibling of the same sex. Or the child may reflect the parents' desires, based on the current composition of the family. Certainly the growing abdominal size of the mother and visible movement of the fetus makes the fetus more concrete and meaningful to all family members, particularly young children. Increased size, though, literally and figuratively increases the distance in the mother-child dyad. This loss of the intense mother-child bond may be felt most acutely by firstborn and only children. The beginnings of the triangle for sibling rivalry are rooted here. The father's relationship with the child can be assessed as a balancing factor. The ability of the the father to adapt during the childbearing cycle to meet the changing needs of the child and perform a wide range of vegetative and nurturing parenting tasks is critical to a healthy outcome.

The family can be assessed for their inclusion of the child in the pregnancy cycle. Has there been an attempt to tell the child about the pregnancy, the growing fetus, or the birth? Has the family acknowledged openly the anxieties and fears a child has about replacement,

Table 3-8. Sibling-Fetal Assessment Areas

Fulfillment of basic individual needs for sibling (food, shelter, clothes, exercise, positive emotional climate, cognitively stimulating environment appropriate to developmental phase)

Parent-child relationship (attachment bonds, communication)

Knowledge and understanding of pregnancy cycle and needs of infant

Differentiation of fetus by sibling (feel fetal movement, fetal parts, gender, awareness of change in abdominal size)

and have they attempted to talk about them? These factors will contribute to the child's positive perception of the pregnancy. Areas for assessment are summarized in Table 3–8.

CHILDBEARING FAMILY SYSTEM ASSESSMENT

Individuals and subsystems comprise the family system, but the family has a life of its own and a relationship to larger systems that all affect the expectant family. The *family* has to achieve certain developmental tasks, aside from its individual members' tasks. First, they must successfully accomplish the tasks necessary to getting themselves established as a family, as this will be important to the outcome of the pregnancy. Following this, their tasks include (1) reevaluating division of labor and responsibility; (2) adapting sexual relations to the pregnant state; (3) adapting relations with extended families; (4) maintaining family members' morale; and (5) preparing for the new family member economically, physically, and emotionally.

In family system assessment, all of the relevant individual data are obtained, plus data relevant to the roles and interactional patterns of the family as a unit (see Table 3–9). Recurring patterns of illness or of social relating are important *historically* as they have been transmitted from one generation to another and may explain and influence current system functioning.

The current family theme is pregnancy; communication, support systems, food, lifestyle, sleep, and emotions all revolve around this pregnant theme and this unborn stranger. The family has to adjust and adapt to this theme because it affects all members. Roles and relationships in the family system must make room for the fetus. Because of the interactional nature of a family system, changes in one person will affect others. During assessment the nurse will monitor the adaptation, flexibility, and problem-solving capabilities of the system as a whole, as it acts to meet the financial, protective, emotional, and physiological demands of childbearing. Particularly important are the family's lifestyle and their ability to make appropriate changes geared toward acquiring a new helpless family member. This requires role flexibility and role evolution in all family members. The ability of a family to make these changes is facilitated by adequate financial and community

Table 3-9. Childbearing Family System Assessment Areas

Family system:
    Communication patterns, including channels and quality of communication, problem solving, decision making, triangling
    Family rules
    Power and authority relations, who makes and enforces rules, methods of discipline employed, who dispenses rewards
    Expectations that family members hold toward one another; clarity
    Family/individual space
    Use of time; recreational and structured time
    Family development phases
    Ascribed and assigned roles within family (e.g., breadwinner, clown, sexual, generational, and functional roles)
    Family lifestyle, including values, recreation, priority tasks, and function
    Health habits and practices, including patterns of nutrition, exercise, and hygiene
    Family resources
    Family role flexibility

Family environment:
    Health care system interaction
    Educational system interaction
    Church involvement
    Employment system interaction
    Cultural influences
    Extended family interaction
    Community activities
    Nonfamily support systems, including friends and neighbors

Multigenerational family information:
    Genogram
    Health history of significant family members
    Occupation
    Relationships; roles
    Family patterns, themes, or diseases (e.g., alcoholism, child abuse)

resources and support systems, that is, a family's closeness to and interactions with the larger system.

The extent to which a family has differentiated itself—that is, developed a variety of functional rules, roles, and patterns of communicating—will be a positive force during pregnancy. Role rigidity and lack of mutually agreed-upon goals or family rules will characterize a less differentiated system. An anticipated change in lifestyle requires that the family closely evaluate family space, resources, priorities, recreational and work patterns, and use of time and health habits.

EXTENDED FAMILY SYSTEM ASSESSMENT

Assessment of the quality and frequency of the interactions with extended family members is important, as old triangles may reemerge during this developmental crisis. Mothers-in-law may be perceived anew as interfering with or monopolizing their sons and daughters. Similarly, there may be renewed and strengthened attempts to transmit multigenerational family values, myths, and processes. Values relating to gender, parenting, and childrearing, may affect the pregnant family positively or may contribute to increased stress.

Since pregnancy is viewed as a developmental crisis, a support network is an important balancing factor, and frequently the extended family provides support through its accumulated knowledge, role modeling, and emotional closeness.

EXTRA SYSTEM LINKAGES

Those nuclear families without a familiar support system need to find supports through friends, church, or community groups or services. A family's openness to reaching out and its ability to initiate relationships and new support systems is important. During the pregnancy phase of family life these new support systems are most helpfully and positively related to pregnancy. Health services, religious and spiritual counseling, educational services focusing on pregnancy and child care and pregnant or childrearing families all constitute typical support networks for the pregnant family. A family with closed, rigid boundaries, isolated from its broader community, is at risk for coping poorly with the pregnancy.

METHODOLOGIES FOR ASSESSMENT

This chapter has dealt so far with what to assess at certain system levels, using some key family system concepts. This section will briefly discuss what methodologies and strategies might be helpful in gathering this broad and sometimes sensitive information. During the assessment process, information is collected from observation and participation in home visits; from interviews with individuals, dyads, and the family as a group; and from health records and other health professionals. Tools that help the nurse organize and conceptualize her collection of data include interview guides, published assessment tools, and the genogram. She examines her data for patterns and for variations from the norm. The analysis of the data leads to diagnosis.

Home Assessment

Nurses usually assess clients in the health care setting, away from the family's natural setting. Although nurses have always been more familar with the homes of their clients than other health professionals, it is really the anthropologists (e.g., Jules Henry, 1973) who have been able to communicate in writing the richness, complexity, and depth that observing a family in their home can hold. Henry, as a result of his intensive daily observations of family patterns, has described manifestations of family pathology around the expression of anger; the use and understanding of food, time, and space in a household; the quality of interpersonal relationships; and the availability of family members to give and receive love. Home visits, which include intensive, consistent observation, attention to detail, and interviewing of all family members, have resulted in an increased understanding of family life that is far richer than clinic interviews could be. Whenever possible, nurses should use this setting to augment their data base. Table 3–10 sets outs some guidelines for home assessment.

Interview

Communication for the purpose of gathering information occurs with the family as individival members and as a unit.Its individual subsystems, its dyads, and extended family members are the basis for the assessment process. Seeing and talking with the system, in parts and as a whole provides the clinician with unique information.

An assessment tool, (which can be developed from materials included in this chapter) to be used during the interview is based on the wholistic framework identified in this chapter and would provide a wealth of material. Interviewing can be broadly based, as in an initial

Table 3-10. Guidelines for Home Assessment of Families,
as Part of the Overall Assessment

Time:
How do individuals and the family as a unit organize their time?
When and for what purposes does family spend time together? Is it task
oriented? Recreational?

Space:
How is space organized?
Is there concern for cleanliness?
Is there space for individual privacy?
Is there adult space and space for children? Family space?
Is care given to the appearance of public and private rooms?
Who uses what space?

Interpersonal communications:
How frequent is interpersonal communication?
Who initiates it?
Who speaks to whom?
What is usually its content?
Is communication clearly spoken and understood?
What is its quality (e.g., laughter, spontaneity, questioning)?

Affect:
How is anger expressed and received?
How is affection expressed and received?

Food:
What is it and how is it served?
Who eats together?

Lifestyle:
What information does the home give about the family's lifestyle (e.g., hobbies and interests such as music, fishing, sports)?

Interaction with community:
How open is the home to the community, through organizational life,
volunteer activities, neighborliness?

assessment, or narrow and intense, aimed at exploring a current timely
area of concern to the family. A formal, structured interview or an informal open-ended approach may be used, depending upon the
circumstances.

Establishing a relationship with the family as a group is an important
nursing intervention in itself, as well as a precursor to collecting reli-

Table 3-11. Ways to Promote Trust
and Facilitate Family Assessment

Avoid judgmental or negative statements.

Maintain interested and friendly communications for all family members.

Maintain good eye contact with all family members.

Consistently enforce structure and rules of interviews, such as keeping appointments promptly, following through with referrals, and letting the family know the time limits of the interview.

Accept communication or other open, nonviolent expression of feelings that are angry, hostile, or positive, without reacting defensively or withdrawing; make a point of asking all family members to express their points of view or feelings.

Express your positive feelings, when appropriate, to family members.

Respond directly, honestly, and openly to family members' queries about diagnosis, medications, need for referrals, and expectations.

Avoid triangling by keeping communication channels open among all family systems, directing communication to the person to whom the message is intended, and avoiding third-party messengers.

Avoid mystification by stating a clear, meaningful message; asking for or giving clarification of intent of message, if necessary; using "I" position statements (e.g., "I am feeling bad about that"); and decoding confusing messages.

Avoid double-bind situations by seeking feedback from sender about which message is really intended, listening to message and clarifying and validating that message; and promoting congruence of affective behavioral components of a message with the verbal content, by verbalizing affective component.

---

able and valid data. Establishing a relationship with the whole family requires a sensitive, thoughtful approach. Since families frequently have subsystem coalitions and alliances, as well as power hierarchies and rules about dealing with outsiders, it is not as simple to form a relationship with the family group as it may appear. The nurse in a physical and interactional sense will promote a relationship with the family by (1) accepting the family lifestyle, the family culture, and alternative family patterns in a nonjudgmental way; (2) promoting open communication with all family members; and (3) expressing positive attitudes and behaviors toward each subsystem member. The family's formation of a bond with an outsider means their boundaries have become both more open and more permeable. The issues involved in promoting trust and thus facilitating assessment are presented in Table 3-11.

Published Tools for Family Assessment

There are several published tools for use in assessment of the family that may be useful for the nurse. Before we discuss some of these, it also should be noted that the literature is full of many small surveys of pregnant families, the data for which were collected by author-developed questionnaires. Nurses may want to use some of those sources as well, or even develop their own tools.

Examples of published family tools include the Family Environment Scale, which is a self-report instrument aimed at measuring the internal environment of a family, tapping 10 relationship, personal-growth, and system-maintenance dimensions: cohesion, expressiveness, conflict, independence, achievement orientation, intellectual cultural orientation, active recreational orientation, moral religious emphasis, organization, and control (Moos & Moos, 1976).

The Card Sort Procedure (Oliveri & Reiss, 1981) is an objective group problem-solving task from which direct measures of family behavior are obtained that are used to obtain estimates of families' characteristic styles of relating to the social environment. These dimensions of family life have been identified as configuration, coordination, and closure. A third example is the Support System Questionnaire, which is used in the assessment of the support system within the family and of significant other support systems. There are rating scales that enable the nurse to evaluate qualitatively and quantitatively a client's perinatal risk status. Based on a client's social, psychological, medical, or obstetrical history, a score is computed that places a woman in a high- or low-risk status category. Many social and psychological factors mentioned in this chaper, (e.g., low income, poor education, deficient support systems) would contribute to a woman's increased risk for poor pregnancy outcome.

CONCLUSION

This chapter has presented a framework for family assessment during the childbearing phase of family life. The framework for assessment has been structured from a systems level perspective and from key concepts drawn from the family systems theory literature.

Unique characteristics of the childbearing family and its members have been described at each system level, using the lens of family concepts. The resulting framework for assessment is clearly a complex and broadly conceived mandate that acknowledges the significance of each family member in the health of the newest developing family member.

REFERENCES

Antle, K. (1975). Psychologic involvement in pregnancy by expectant fathers. *Journal of Obstetric, Gynecologic & Neonatal Nursing, 4*, 40–42.

Bowen, M. (1978). *Family theory in clinical practice*. New York: Jason Aronson.

Brazelton, T. B. (1973). Effect of maternal expectations on early infant behavior. *Early Child Development Care, 2*, 259–273.

Broom, B. (1984). Consensus about the marital relationship during transition to parenthood. *Nursing Research, 334*, 223–228.

Caplan, G. (1960). Patterns of paternal response to the crisis of premature birth. *Psychiatry, 23*, 365–374.

Erikson, E. (1963). *Childhood and society* (2nd ed.). New York: W. W. Norton.

Hartman, A. A., & Nicolay, R. C. (1966). Sexual deviant behavior in expectant fathers. *Journal of Abnormal Psychology, 71*, 233–243.

Henry, J. (1973). *Pathways to madness*. New York: Vintage.

Herzog, J. M. (1982). Patterns of expectant fatherhood: A study of the fathers of a group of premature infants. In S. Cahn, N. Gurwitt, & J. M. Ross (Eds.), *Father and child*. Boston: Little, Brown.

Hobbs, D. F., & Cole, S. P. (1976). Transition to parenthood: A decade replication. *Journal of Marriage and the Family, 38*, 723–731.

Hott, J. R. (1976). The crisis of expectant fatherhood. *American Journal of Nursing*, 1436–1440.

Jiminez, M., & Newton, N. (1982). Job orientation and adjustment to pregnancy and early motherhood. *Birth, 9*, 157–160.

Lamb, G., & Lipkin, M. (1982). Somatic symptoms of expectant fathers. *MCN, The Journal of Maternal-Child Nursing, 7*, 110–115.

Leonard, S. (1976). How first time fathers feel toward their newborns. *MCN, The Journal of Maternal-Child Nursing, 1*, 361–365.

Marquart, R. K. (1976). Expectant fathers: What are their needs? *MCN, The Journal of Maternal-Child Nursing, 1*, 32–37.

May, K. (1982). The father as observer. *MCN, The Journal of Maternal-Child Nursing, 7*, 319–322.

Miller, S., & Winstead-Fry, P. (1982). *Family systems theory in nursing practice*. Reston, VA: Reston Publishing.

Moos, R., & Moos, B. (1976). A typology of family social environments. *Family Process, 15*, 357–372.

Obzrut, L. A. (1976). Expectant fathers' perceptions of fathering. *American Journal of Nursing*, 1440–1442.

Oliveri, M., & Reiss, O. (1981). A theory based empirical classification of family problem-solving behavior. *Family Process, 20*, 409–418.

Pendagast, E., & Sherman, C. (1978). A guide to the genogram family system training. *The Family, 5,* 3-5.

Reiber, V. (1976). Is the nuturing role natural to fathers? *MCN, The Journal of Maternal-Child Nursing, 1,* 366-371.

Rubin, R. (1967). Attainment of the maternal role, part 1: Processes. *Nursing Research, 16,* 237-245.

Rubin, R. (1972). Fantasy and object constancy in maternal relations. *MCN, The Journal of Maternal-Child Nursing, 1,* 101-111.

Rubin, R. (1975). Maternal tasks in pregnancy. *MCN, The Journal of Maternal-Child Nursing, 4,* 143-153.

Russell, C. S. (1974). Transition to parenthood: Problems and gratifications. *Journal of Marriage and the Family, 36,* 294-301.

Satir, V. (1967). *Conjunct family therapy.* Palo Alto, CA: Science and Behavior Books.

Sherwen, L. (1981). Fantasies during the third trimester of pregnancy. *MCN, The Journal of Maternal-Child Nursing, 6,* 398-401.

Trethowan, W. H., & Conlon, M. F. (1965). The couvade syndrome. *British Journal of Psychiatry, 111,* 57-66.

Wandersman, L., Wandersman, A., & Kahn, S. (1980). Social support in the transition to parenthood. *Journal of Community Psychology, 8,* 332-342.

Chapter 4

Sexuality and Sex Roles in the Pregnant Family

Until recently, the sexual dimension of the pregnant family was the aspect most frequently ignored or glossed over by nurses and other primary caretakers. While still not a teaching and counseling area with which most professionals feel great comfort, nurses and others have accepted responsibility for talking with pregnant couples who are concerned with their sexuality. The majority of literature emerging from behavioral and nursing research that deals with sexuality during pregnancy speaks to changes in sexual behaviors throughout the course of the three trimesters. Nurses may use such information to point out possible changes in feelings and behaviors a couple may experience as pregnancy progresses. Moreover, suggestions might be made to the couple based on these trends, in an effort to maximize sexual pleasure during this time.

A major drawback to much literature concerned with sex during pregnancy, however, is the focus on the purely functional aspects of sexual behaviors, that is, its cognitive, physical, and emotional aspects. A systems perspective mandates that, where a function exists, a structure within the system will underlie its manifestation. Further, the structure and function of human sexuality may lie at two system levels, that of the individual system and that of the family system.

It becomes evident that the concept of human sexuality is a very complex one, even without the extra complexities introduced by pregnancy. In its most basic sense, sexuality may be considered as a part of human identity. Sexual identity of members of the family system will foster certain distinct patterns of interaction in the family. Depending on the underlying sexual structure of the family members and the pattern of sexual interactions within the family, the family during pregnancy will function in a variety of ways. These functions are the behaviors identified in the literature concerned with sex during pregnancy. To gain an appreciation and understanding of such sexual behaviors, the nurse must first consider the family sexual structure and, what is even more basic, the sexual structure of the individual members.

The fundamental question remains: What is sexual identity in the human system, and how will it come to direct the sexual function of the family system during pregnancy? Nass, Libby, and Fisher (1983) see sexuality and sexual identity as pervading all aspects of the human individual. Sexual identity is concerned with the biological, sociological, spiritual, and cultural aspects of life. Further, it is intrinsic to the concept of human identity. Human identity can be divided into components including ethnic, age, job, family, religious, social class, political, and sexual identity. Sexual identity can be further broken down into biological aspects, social gender role (sex-role identity), sexual preference, body image, and sexual scripts. For purposes of this chapter, we will be mainly concerned with biological sexual aspects and social gender role or orientation in the individual and the ramifications of such individual sexual identity for the pregnant family system.

PSYCHOSEXUAL DEVELOPMENT

Before an individual can function as a sexual entity in a family, he or she must develop a sexual identity. As mentioned earlier, development of sexuality or a sexual identity in the individual is part of the more encompassing process of child growth and development. Unfortunately, terms such as *sexuality, sexual identity, sex role,* and so on are often used interchangeably by different theorists. In addition, the nature of hypotheses concerning evolution of sexual identity differ, depending upon the theoretical orientation of the theorist discussing such development. In this chapter, the term *sexual identity* will be used to refer to the broad sexual sphere of the individual system, encompassing sexual structure or makeup (biological, psychosocial, and cultural) and the function of that structure through sexual behaviors.

There are many theories of psychosexual development. It is not within the scope of this book to discuss them all in depth. Three frequently cited theories will be briefly mentioned by way of examples of psychosocial development that may be expected to impact on the structure and function of the pregnant family.

Psychoanalytic Theory

Formulated by Freud and others, this theory is of concern, since it is the only theory of human development that accords sexuality a place of paramount importance (Katchadourian & Lunde, 1972). This formulation begins with the assumption that each newborn human starts out with a certain amount of sexual (libidinal) energy. Psychosexual development is the process by which the libidinal energy is invested in zones of the body found to be pleasurable to the human system at successive stages of the life cycle. The sequence of investment is not random, but follows a definite pattern which is coordinated with physiological maturation (Bemporad, 1980; Stream, 1983). These well-known stages are the oral, anal, phallic, latency, and genital stages. The highest level of psychosexual development is attainment of the genital stage, which signals attainment of a mature sexual identity. This level of psychosexual development integrates all earlier levels and facilitates establishment of satisfactory life patterns of sex, procreation, and work (Bemporad, 1980; Katchadourian & Lunde, 1972).

Erikson's Psychosocial Theory

Building on the psychoanalytic base, Erikson evolved his "epigenetic" theory of personality, which expands the concept of psychosexual development. While agreeing that at specific stages in a human system's ontogeny, some particular function reaches special importance and that an appropriate environmental response is necessary for normal growth, Erikson expands the psychoanalytic concept and defines such stages as times of crisis in which the individual's innate level of maturation encounters conflicts with social mores. In a further expansion of theory, Erikson attempts to describe how the child is viewed by the self and others during these stages. A listing of Erikson's well-known stages of development that relate to sexual maturity and the stage of Freudian psychosexual development that each parallels follows (Bemporad, 1980; Stream, 1983):

Eriksonian Stage	Freudian Stage
Trust vs. mistrust	Oral
Autonomy vs. shame and doubt	Anal
Initiative vs. guilt	Phallic-Oedipal
Industry vs. inferiority	Latency
Identity vs. identity diffusion	Genital

Using these two theories to complement each other gives a much broader view of the psychological and social processes involved in an individual's becoming a mature sexual being.

Learning Theory

The final theory concerned with psychosexual development in the individual system to be briefly considered here is learning theory. In this perspective, combined sexual learnings (which occur through a series of spontaneous discoveries) and positive and negative reinforcements (pleasure and parental disapproval) evolve into a learned sexual orientation for each individual. This learned sexual orientation produces a human system with an identifiable sexual structure and functions (behaviors) (Katchadourian & Lunde, 1972). These individual structures affect sexual structure in the family system and will be one determinant of sexual function during pregnancy.

SEXUAL STRUCTURE IN THE FAMILY SYSTEM

Through the mechanisms just discussed or other mechanisms, the human individual develops a sexual identity—all that she or he is as a sexual being. Sexual identity does not evolve in a vacuum, however, but in the family of origin. The manifestation of sexuality also does not occur in a vacuum, but in a group. The group that we are concerned with here is the nuclear family of procreation, specifically during the childbearing phase. Each individual, male and female, upon establishing a new family unit, will bring along a sexual structure—his or her sexual identity. In the family system, mutual interactions will occur and be influenced by the individual's innate sexual identity. Thus, the action moves to a different system level in the hierarchy—that of the family. One of the primary ways family sexuality is demonstrated is through sex roles and associated norms, and the functions role players perform in the family system. These roles determine manifestations of all sexual behavior, including that occurring during the phase of pregnancy.

SEX ROLES AND THEIR DYNAMICS IN THE FAMILY SYSTEM

Zuengler and Neubeck (1983) discuss the "roots" of sexuality in the family system and identify these roots as family roles and the rules and myths surrounding these roles. The defining of sex roles (behaviors, attitudes, and feelings expected of females and males) is seen as a primary way of teaching sexual behavior and attitudes within the family. Behavior and expectations are governed according to gender in many aspects of our lives, as children incorporate parental messages of what constitutes feminine or masculine behavior. Once learned in the family of origin, sex roles and associated expectations of what someone in a sex role will do tend to remain, to some extent, throughout the individual's life.

Associated with sex roles are certain rules for interacting as a sexual being within a family. Rules may be overt or covert, but they prove to be a very effective means of passing on attitudes concerned with sexuality. An example of an overt rule, stated in the family, might be that a daughter not be allowed to date until she is 16 years of age. A covert rule, on the other hand, may be a silent prohibition for same-sexed family members to touch or kiss. These rules state explicit expectations concerning behaviors of males and females in a particular family system.

Another factor concerning behavior in a sex role within the family is defined by Zuengler and Neubeck (1983) as the family "myths" concerning sexuality. These myths are defined as "accounts" of family sexual behavior, which affect expectations of the self and other family members. An example might be, "All the men in this family are womanizers." Such a myth may be hard to live up to, for the child in a masculine role. Violation of the myths can engender guilt in the individual who transgresses, making that person feel she or he is not living up to the role in the family's eyes. Thus, sex roles are learned in a family system and often determine what we will bring to our family of procreation.

Feldman's (1982) well-documented analysis of sex roles and family dynamics provides some conclusions concerning the function of sex roles in the family that are highly relevant here. According to Feldman, there are two domains for behaviors associated with sex roles: psychological and social. Feldman first identifies the psychological domain of the sex role by specifying characteristics of the male or female personality that have been gleaned from the literature and represent the psychological dimensions of male and female roles. "Feminine" psychological role expectations for women include such adjectives as home and children oriented, warm, affectionate, gentle, tender, empathic, considerate, tactful, compassionate, moody, excitable, emotional, subjective, illogical, complaining, weak, helpless, fragile, easily emotionally hurt, submissive, yielding and dependent. "Masculine" psychological expectations for men include ambitious, competitive, enterprising, worldly, calm, stable, unemotional, realistic, logical, strong, tough, powerful, aggressive, forceful, decisive, dominant, independent, self-reliant, harsh, stern, cruel, autocratic, rigid, arrogant, and so on. These "feminine" and "masculine" adjectives are usually used by individuals in describing a woman or man in a particular sex role. Individuals also often use them to describe themselves, thus giving clues to their sex role identity.

Feldman (1982) divides the sociological domain for sex-role expectations into three categories: economic providing, housework, and childcare. The literature again defines normative behaviors associated with the masculine and feminine roles. For example, concerning economic providing, there is a clear expectation in our society that the man should assume the major share of this responsibility. Even when the woman works outside the home, her job is usually seen as supplemental to the man's job. There is still, in fact, strong social disapproval for the man not working outside the home. In the area of housework, the expectation is that women, even when both spouses work outside the home, maintain the major responsibility. This is an expectation maintained not only by men, but also supported by women. The norm for childcare is similar to that of housework, but to a lesser degree. Even though a 1976 study by Nye (1976) indicated that a majority of husbands and wives felt a father should be involved in childcare, the type of care to be delivered by each role differed. Women were seen as responsible for nurturing, caretaking activities, and men, for "protective" activities (Feldman, 1982). Such a finding has great importance when we consider the current trend to involve fathers in pregnancy and in nurturing their newborn infants. It is apparent that, despite the effects of the woman's movement, many residual stereotypic dimensions of the masculine and feminine roles remain.

Feldman (1982) then constructs several hypotheses concerning the relationship of the sex roles, and their associated psychological and sociological expectations, to three areas of family dynamics: marital interaction, parent-child interaction, and sanctions. These hypotheses bear direct relevance for the family system during pregnancy.

Marital Interaction and Sex Roles

Feldman (1982) proposes two hypotheses concerning the relationship between sex roles and marital interaction:

1. Sex-role conditioning will have a negative influence on both marital intimacy and problem solving. This will occur by inhibiting certain forms of behavior in men and women. The behaviors men will inhibit will be emotional expressiveness, emotional empathy, and mature dependency. Women will inhibit instrumental behavior, assertiveness, and mature independence.
2. Sex-role expectations promote certain dysfunctional attitudes and behaviors in men and women. These will also have a negative effect on intimacy and problem solving in the family system. For women, the main behaviors developed are nagging and pressuring; for men, passive-aggressive behavior and physical violence.

An extrapolation from Feldman's (1982) reported research which identified psychological and sociological characteristics of the masculine and feminine sex roles makes both hypotheses seem logical.

In the marital system, masculine and feminine sex roles act in a synergistic and mutually reinforcing way. Role expectations and their resulting behaviors will interact with each other, and in turn, reinforce each other in an ongoing family cycle of behavior (Feldman, 1982). Feldman identifies several such areas of marital interaction where sex role characteristics "key-in" and reinforce each other, often to the detriment of the family dynamics. One area is sexual behavior (i.e., sexual activities). Sex role expectations tend to make the woman passive in her sexual interactions. Assertive sexuality is seen as undesirable as part of the feminine sex role. The man, according to sex-role expectations, is active and aggressive in pursuing sexual activity. Further, there is little role expectation that he be empathic regarding his partner's needs. The two sets of role behaviors key in to each other. The woman's inhibitions regarding sexual assertiveness prevent her from making advances, which reinforces the man's concept of her lack of interest in sex. This, in turn, reinforces his inhibition of attempting to meet his partner's sexual needs, which will further inhibit her expression of those needs. The dynamic, circular interaction and feedback pattern is evident.

A second area in marital relations where sex roles exert an influence is in the expression of independence and dependence in the family. Here, women expect to be emotionally and financially dependent on men, and men expect to be emotionally and financially independent. These behaviors "fit" together and will further inhibit mature dependency in men and mature independence in women. Again, a mutually reinforcing interaction pattern is evolved.

Marital conflict is a third area where Feldman (1982) sees the effects of sex roles. They influence the frequency and intensity of forms of conflict, and they interfere with problem solving. One important form of conflict seen in marriage is lack of communication. In this instance, the feminine sex-role orientation tends to make the woman overexpressive, while a masculine sex role orientation makes the man underexpressive. Again, these characteristics produce a dynamic feedback loop, reinforcing the pattern. When the couple engages in problem-solving activities, sex-role expectations can produce a masculine role that inhibits emotional expressiveness and empathy and fosters physical violence. The feminine role inhibits assertiveness and instrumental negotiation behaviors and asserts emotional pressuring. The man's lack of expressiveness and understanding stimulates an emotional overreaction in the woman, which negatively impacts problem-solving behaviors.

Parent-Child Interaction and Sex Roles

The following are Feldman's (1982) hypotheses concerning the influence of sex roles on parent-child interaction:

1. Sex-role expectations will exert a negative influence on parent-child interaction by inhibiting certain forms of behavior in the mother and father. Mothers tend to inhibit behaviors associated with parental authority and discipline. Fathers inhibit expressive and nurturing behaviors.
2. Sex-role expectations promote dysfunctional attitudes and behaviors in mothers and fathers that interfere with constructive, growth-promoting parenting. For mothers, the behaviors manifested are overprotectiveness and overcontrol; for fathers, authoritarianism and rigidity.

As with marital interaction, masculine and feminine sex roles interact and mutually reinforce each other in terms of parenting children. The two areas of family function in respect to care of children said to be affected by sex-role typing here are parental authority and discipline, and nurturance and involvement. The inhibition of parental authority in women keys into masculine sex-role expectations that promote rigid authoritarianism in men. The inhibition of involvement and nurturance of children among men promotes the feminine role of great involvement and nurturance, which can lead a woman to be overinvolved and overprotective of her children. Again, these behavioral patterns will reinforce one another, creating a cyclical dynamic.

Sanctions and Sex Roles

The final area dealt with by Feldman (1982) concerning effects of sex-roles on family dynamics is the sanctions designed to maintain the family patterns as they are. His hypothesis concerned with sanctions states that sex-role-congruent attitudes and behaviors will be maintained by positive sanctions (rewards) and negative sanctions (punishment) for role conformity. Both positive and negative sanctions may be externally generated by others, and internally generated by the self. Approval and disapproval from others external to the family unit, as

well as intrapsychic reactions, (anxiety, silence) are strong reinforcements that assure sex-role conformity.

Feldman (1982) summarizes his formulations concerning sex roles
and family dynamics by citing the major problem with narrowly
defined sex roles. He feels that sex roles promote development of rigid
family systems. These rigid systems and the individuals caught within
them are limited in their capacity to adapt to changing circumstances.

Androgyny: The Alternative to Masculine and Feminine Sex Roles

Androgyny is a concept that evolved during the 1970s and provides
an alternative model to adoption of the masculine and feminine sex
roles previously discussed. Androgyny is of two types, psychological
and sociological. Bem (1975), one of the primary researchers and
theoreticians of the concept of psychological androgyny, describes it as
a state of affairs in which individuals experience the psychological
freedom to develop both the masculine and feminine aspects of their
personalities. Further, the individual will engage in behaviors that contain both masculine and feminine qualities, according to the demands
of the situation and the nature of the individual (Bem, 1974).

Sociological androgyny, on the other hand, describes a state of affairs in which the allocation of work and family responsibility is based
on individual preference and capability, not gender (Feldman, 1982).
In terms of family system dynamics, individuals would interact in a
flexible manner, freed from sex-role limitations on behavior. Such
flexible interactions have been postulated to have beneficial effects for
family functioning as a whole.

Research has demonstrated mixed results concerning the benefits of
maintaining an androgynous role orientation. Generally, researchers
have demonstrated that androgynous individuals are more flexible
and adaptive than sex-typed individuals (Bem, 1975; Bem & Lenny,
1976; Osofsky & Windle, 1978; Wiggins & Holzmuller, 1981). There is
also evidence that androgynous individuals who perceive equality in
male and female dyadic interactions have an increased satisfaction
with sexual behaviors and relations (Hatfield, Greenberger, Traupmann, & Lambert, 1982; Safir, 1982). Feldman and Aschenbrenner
(1983) have identified a shift in role qualities of androgynous couples
during the course of pregnancy, with both men and women increasing

in "female" role behavior and instrumental personality traits. This seems to demonstrate an appropriate response to specific circumstances—pregnancy and parenthood.

Several investigators, however, have found that androgynous individuals do not have the highest level of mental health. Whitney (1983), after a meta-analysis of 35 studies, found that there was a relationship between a masculine sex-role orientation and self-esteem (when both men and women were included in the samples). Bessoff and Glass (1982), in another meta-analysis of data from 26 studies, found a strong positive association between a masculine sex-role orientation and mental health. Finally, Lenz, Soeken, Rankin, and Fishmen (1985) found that a couple's femininity score, and not their androgyny score, was positively correlated to perceptions of the quality of the marital relationship in the postpartum period.

Research into social androgyny has been very scarce. Since sociological androgyny implies a flexible, open social system in which women and men participate in both provider and nurturer roles, one would expect some change in parenting behaviors. These might or might not be beneficial to the child. Theoretically, since androgynous individuals tend to be more flexible, adaptive, and competent, one might postulate that parenting behaviors would also be more flexible, adaptive, and competent. Baumrind (1982) investigated parents of 78 female and 86 male 9-year-old children. She found that, while androgynous women did not differ from feminine sex-role-typed women in their childrearing practices, androgynous men were more like androgynous women than masculine men in this regard. Androgynous parents were also more likely to be "child centered" in their approach to parenting than sex-role-typed parents. However, Baumrind also found that children of sex-role-typed parents tended to be more competent than children of androgynous parents, and so cautioned professionals against prematurely proclaiming androgyny as the new ideal for family role functions.

SEX-ROLE DYNAMICS IN THE PREGNANT FAMILY

If we examined the sex-role hypotheses of Feldman (1982) and the function of the androgynous role in families, some hypotheses might be made concerning the function of these roles during pregnancy. We will consider three situations: sex-typed (masculine and feminine) roles during pregnancy; androgynous roles during pregnancy; and internal and external sanctions on the pregnant couple to maintain certain behaviors during pregnancy.

Masculine and Feminine Sex Roles during Pregnancy

Sexual Interactions. While each partner in many young couples may equally initiate sexual behaviors in their early dyadic relationship, this pattern has been shown to alter during pregnancy (Woods & Dery, 1984). For a variety of reasons, both physical and psychological, the woman often loses sexual interest during the first trimester. She may fall into a feminine sex-role pattern of great passivity and even rejection of her mate's sexual advances. The man perceives his mate's increasing sexual passivity and feels he should initiate sexual activity. Because of his feelings concerning his mate's pregnancy, however, he cannot even function in a truly masculine role-stereotypic way without guilt. This feeling may continue throughout the pregnancy, even during the second trimester, when some women demonstrate increased sexual desire. The need to be sexually assertive to meet the mate's passivity and reluctance in the first and third trimesters may take the man outside the home for sexual relations, a trend supported by the literature (Osofsky & Osofsky, 1980). Finally, for the man, falling into a masculine sex-role pattern may make him less empathic to his pregnant mate's needs and less willing to attempt to meet them in alternative pleasuring patterns often suggested by health care professionals.

Dependence and Independence. During pregnancy, the tendency for a woman in a "feminine" role is to become even more dependent on her mate. Caplan (1959) describes clearly the introversion, self-centeredness, passivity, dependence, and emotional lability experienced as pregnancy progresses. Thus, the feminine role-typed woman, who perceives herself as emotionally and financially dependent on her mate in the first place, may experience an increase in these feelings during pregnancy.

Meanwhile, the man in a masculine-type role believes he should be emotionally independent. He is not prepared for the emotional conflicts he feels during pregnancy. Men also have been found to experience the need for mothering and attention, in short, the need to have dependency needs met (Caplan, 1959). This need to be dependent may make him feel guilty. He may further resent his mate's increased dependence on him, and, since he has unmet dependency needs himself, he may be totally unable to give his mate the support she needs. Again, he may retreat from the situation, either physically or emotionally, or seek elsewhere to have his own needs met, since his mate will not be able to nurture him.

Conflict Resolution and Communication. The scenario described by Feldman (1982) concerning conflict resolution and communication patterns among individuals in sex-typed roles is likely to be exaggerated during pregnancy.

First, the woman, seen as tending toward overexpressiveness, will be experiencing emotional lability and mood swings. Her expressiveness or overexpressiveness may take on a totally irrational character, little related to external events or causes. The woman's mate is doubly confused, since he cannot understand or deal with the nature of his mate's expressions and, further, he may be experiencing emotional turmoil himself. If he adheres to a masculine-typed role pattern, he will see himself as the strong, silent type and suppress his feelings, not communicating them at all to his mate. Meanwhile, the woman continues to communicate, perhaps in excess, her newly experienced moods and concerns. Since the man is so often confused by his mate's moods and cannot understand her communications and further feels he can't tell her about his own emotional state, it is possible that his empathy for his mate will decrease. His feelings of anger and aggression may increase, directed toward his mate, the pregnancy, the fetus, or all three.

This block in communication and empathy between the man and woman in sex-typed roles may be a special disadvantage during pregnancy. This is a time when, due to the progression of the pregnancy, typical role behaviors may need to be altered to maintain family function. For example, due to fatigue and nausea, the woman may be unable to do housework. She would like to negotiate with her mate and have him assume some of her responsibilities around the house. These activities are viewed by the man as "woman's work." Blocked communication and decreased empathy may make adjustment of role responsibilities impossible to negotiate for the couple, and marital discord may develop.

Parenting. The man adhering to a masculine-typed role may believe that he should not be involved in care of his infant-to-be. Emotionally, however, he may desire more involvement with the pregnancy and future infant but believes these emotions are weak and inappropriate. He may therefore reluctantly withdraw from the idea of future involvement with his newborn.

The woman in a feminine-typed role would agree that her mate has no role in nurturing the newborn; that this is her area of expertise and he is not allowed to participate. Even if her mate plans to become involved with the newborn, or plans involvement during the pregnancy, the woman may discourage him in many ways. Any attempts at the father's becoming involved in nurturing the infant may be effectively sabotaged by his mate.

Androgynous Role Patterns during Pregnancy

While avoiding the view that androgyny is the panacea for parenting and marital problems, it would seem that couples with an androgynous orientation may have an easier time adjusting to pregnancy. Since both the man and woman are free to express masculine and feminine behaviors, there would be no prohibition to the father communicating his wants and needs concerning the pregnancy to his mate. Further, negotiations concerning role responsibilities in the area of housework and plans for childcare would be easier. It would be no "disgrace" for the father to assume responsibility for housework or desire involvement with nurturing the newborn.

While pregnancy, especially the first, is still fraught with conflicts and potential problems, it would seem that a more flexible attitude to what is appropriate role behavior would greatly assist with resolution of conflicts that occur in all families during pregnancy.

External Sanctions on the Pregnant Couple

In the previous discussion of areas of family dynamics during pregnancy, some aspects of the internal sanctions that compel an individual to fulfill sex-typed role behaviors were mentioned. Guilt and a feeling that behavior is inappropriate are primary internal sanctions. External sanctions may be far more problematic for the couple, as they may be more ambiguous, and conflicting messages may come from different sources in the couple's world.

Many health care professionals, and especially nurses, behave toward pregnant couples as if we assume that they all have an androgynous role orientation. We assume that all men want to be involved in the pregnancy, to be present and active at labor and delivery, and actively to nurture the infant. We further assume that all women want the father's involvement. This may not be so for individuals adhering to a more traditional sex role. Our pressuring couples to adopt behavior that they see as inappropriate may increase their feelings of guilt and conflict. They may feel like they are "bad parents" or may get the message that professionals don't believe they want to do what's best for their child.

On the other hand, it is highly possible that couples with an androgynous orientation get many negative messages from extended families. A couple's parents were probably reared into more rigidly defined sex roles; to these parents, the behaviors of their offspring may seem totally inappropriate to them. They then communicate negative messages concerning these androgynous behaviors, and the pregnant couple may again experience guilt or believe they are behaving in an inappropriate pattern.

It might seem highly appropriate, then, for nurses and other health care professionals to ascertain how the pregnant partners perceive their respective roles, before advocating any one course of action or behavior. Just as masculine and feminine roles may not work for everyone, so might androgynous roles not work for some women and men as well.

SEXUAL BEHAVIOR IN THE PREGNANT FAMILY

Much attention in this chapter has been directed toward the structure of sexuality in the family system, especially during pregnancy. What does the literature indicate concerning the functional aspects of sexuality in the pregnant family? Are there any trends that can be identified?

In general, an investigation of literature indicates that different studies have used greatly different designs, methodologies, samples, assessments, and analysis techniques. It thus becomes difficult to define a specific "trend" in sexual behaviors during pregnancy. The major pattern found consistently throughout the studies is a decline in sexual interest and behavior of women during the third trimester. Changes in sexuality during the earlier stages of pregnancy are far less clearly established (Calhoun, Selby, & King, 1981). In addition, many investigators postulate that behaviors of women during pregnancy are affected by complex and changing psychological and physiological factors (Masters & Johnson, 1966; White & Reamy, 1982). Their mate's behaviors are also mediated by psychological factors (Osofsky, 1982). A closer look at sexual patterns for women during each trimester and men during pregnancy in general will give a clearer picture of sexual behavior in the pregnant family.

The Mother-to-Be

First Trimester. Investigators report different findings concerning a woman's sexual behaviors during the first trimester. Masters and Johnson (1966) found, in their sample, a great variation in levels of eroticism and levels of sexual performance. In terms of physiological changes during the first trimester, Masters and Johnson feel that breast tenderness, nausea, sleepiness, and chronic fatigue affect sexual function. Kenney (1973) looked at sexual desire, frequency, enjoyment, and orgasm in a sample of 33 women. In the first trimester, he found little difference in these indicators of sexual function from prepregnant levels. Falicov (1973) defined sexual function somewhat differently, in terms of frequency of coitus, degree of sexual interest and feelings of eroticism, and sexual satisfaction. In his sample of 19 primiparas, all subjects had experienced a moderate to marked decline in these variables by the end of the first trimester. Factors affecting this response included physiological symptoms of nausea, vomiting, heartburn, and somatic complaints related to sexual function (i.e., feeling the vagina was smaller or numb). The main psychological factor affecting sexual function during the first trimester in Falicov's sample was fear of hurting the fetus.

Tolor and DiGranzia (1976) obtained different findings with a sample of 216 women. They found that women during the first trimester differed little from the prepregnant level in their preference for sexual relations and satisfaction with the rate of sexual activity. In contrast with these findings are those of Battacchi (1978), who sampled 500 pregnant women relative to three aspects of sexual function: satisfaction, frequency of coitus, and libido. During the first trimester, a large number of women noted a decrease in these parameters (satisfaction, 36%; frequency, 44.6%; libido, 28.2%), as compared to those noting an increase (satisfaction, 10.4%; frequency, 8.2%; libido, 10.2%). In a sample of 119 women, Robson, Brant, and Kumar (1981) reported that only 7 women in the sample reported an increase in frequency of intercourse in the first trimester.

As can be seen, while study results are mixed and indicators of sexual function are not consistent from study to study, some decrease in sexual function is noted across most studies during the first trimester. Physiological and psychological factors are implicated in these changes.

Second Trimester. Many investigators found a shift, in at least some of their subjects, toward increased sexual interest and activity during the second trimester. Masters and Johnson (1966) found an increase in eroticism and effectiveness of sexual performance, well above what was experienced in the nonpregnant state, during this time. Possible changes in physiology related to this finding may be the increased vascularity of pelvic viscera and an awareness of increased sexual tension occurring in the early part of the second trimester.

Findings of both Kenny (1973) and Falicov (1973) disagree with those of Masters and Johnson (1966) concerning sexuality in the second trimester. While Falicov (1973) did find that second trimester coital frequency and sexual satisfaction did increase above levels of the first trimester, they still remained far below prepregnancy levels. Factors accounting for the finding during the second trimester were tiredness, breast tenderness, and genital discomfort. The enlarging abdomen made modification of coital position necessary for some women. Psychologically, women still feared harming the fetus, but not as intensely. Kenny (1973), in contrast, found no difference in sexual function between the first and second trimester, both being at a level similar to the prepregnant period.

Tolor and DiGranzia (1976) found that women in the second trimester were as satisfied with their current rate of sexual activity as women in the first trimester. There was also a significantly greater incidence of multiple orgasm in women in their second trimester in this investigation. Lumley (1978), while finding that the frequency of sexual intercourse declined progressively from the first to the third trimesters, did note an increase in libido and coital frequency during the second trimester for 11% of his sample (N=26).

Returning to Battacchi's (1978) study of three aspects of sexuality (satisfaction, frequency, and libido), we find an increase in the proportion of women reporting improvement in the three indicators (satisfaction, 12.6%; frequency, 10.6%; and libido, 14.2%) over levels of the first trimester. Finally, Robson and associates (1981) found a similar pattern of increased frequency of intercouse between the first and second trimester.

The pattern of sexual behavior is seen to vary greatly with each investigator. Sexual pleasure and frequency are seen to increase in some studies and to stay the same as in the first trimester in others. No consensus may be reached among current investigators concerning sexual behavior during the second trimester.

Third Trimester. During the third trimester, most investigators confirm a decrease in sexual activity and desire. Masters and Johnson (1966) note a significant decrease in sexual activity in both parous and nulliparous women during the last trimester. Women reported a decrease in sexual interest and more somatic complaints, including pelvic tension and backache. During orgasm, spasm of the uterus was observed for as long as one minute. While these physiological complaints may have been involved in the decreased activity, Masters and Johnson also noted that many of the women in their sample had been warned by their physicians not to have intercourse for periods of four weeks to three months before delivery.

Other investigators report similar findings. Kenny (1973) described a decrease in coital frequency, desire, and enjoyment but found that orgasm remained the same. He suggests considering pregnancy, as it relates to sexual activity, in two phases for future research: the last six weeks and the entire first part of pregnancy.

Falicov's (1973) subjects reported fluctuations in sexual desire during the third trimester. By the eighth month, the majority of his sample had discontinued sexual intercourse. Tolor and DiGranzia (1976) found some inconsistency in their sample in women's reported satisfaction with the rate of sexual activity. In the third trimester, women were dissatisfied with the rate of intercourse, either desiring more or less sexual activity. There was also a reported lack of multiple orgasms during the third trimester and a progressive decline in sexual interest levels.

Battacchi (1978) found a large drop in the proportion of women reporting an improvement in their sexual functioning during the third trimester (satisfaction,3.0%; frequency,2.6%; and libido, 8.2%). Concomitantly, a large proportion of women in the sample noted a major decrease in the three parameters during the third trimester (satisfaction, 73%; frequency, 85%; and libido, 52.2%). Finally, Robson et al. (1981), in their sample of 119 women, found that by the third trimester, only 40% of the women still found intercourse pleasurable.

Clearly, the trend in the third trimester is toward decreased pleasure and/or interest in sex and increased somatic complaints that affect sexual behavior.

The Father-to Be

Research concerning the father-to-be's sexual behavior during his mate's pregnancy is almost totally lacking. Studies and theory concerning the father's sexual response during pregnancy may be divided into research on sexual function and on the psychological effects of a mate's pregnancy on the man.

Selby and Calhoun (1981), in a study of 25 couples, found that men reported an increase in sexual desire over the course of the pregnancy but a decrease in sexual behavior. Osofsky (1982), using a case-study approach, found that men during pregnancy reported increased sexual problems.

In addition, several psychological factors emerge from this literature that may affect the man's sexual functioning. Included are generally unfounded fears of hurting their wives and unborn babies, uneasiness over having intercourse with a pregnant woman, dislike (or like) of the pregnant body, fear of starting labor or uterine contractions with the mate's orgasm, fantasies of relationships and affairs with other women (or actual affairs), blurring of the mate with a man's mother, and homosexual fantasies (Dameron, 1983; Osofsky & Osofsky, 1980; White & Reamy, 1982). It can be seen that much additional research into a father-to-be's sexual feelings and behaviors is necessary before drawing any conclusions on the subject.

Other Factors That Affect Sexual Function in the Pregnant Family

A variety of variables have been shown to alter the sexual behaviors of a couple during pregnancy. Among these are the increased need for closeness (Tolor & DiGranzia, 1976), perception of the pregnant body (body image), cultural norms for pregnancy, views held by the couple concerning motherhood, and function of the marital dyad (Osofsky & Osofsky, 1980; Woods & Dery, 1984). Many of these areas will be discussed in other chapters, so they will merely be mentioned here. It is important for the reader to keep in mind, however, that all variables concerning the pregnant family are interrelated and affect each other.

NURSING ASSESSMENT AND INTERVENTION WITH THE PREGNANT FAMILY

In contemplating nursing activities to assist women and men in adjusting to a changed sex life during pregnancy, it is necessary to use the broad perspective of sexual structure and function in the family. The pregnant woman and her mate will be experiencing changes not only in sexual desire and behavior but also in their patterns of sex roles and role interactions. Both realms may prove problematic for the couple and may impede smooth functioning of the family unit in general.

Model for Sexuality Intervention

Mims and Swenson (1980) provide a useful model for sexuality intervention which has relevance for our discussion of structure and function of sexuality in the pregnant family. The model is composed of four hierarchical levels designed to provide nurses with direction for interaction with clients. The first and lowest level is the *life experience* level, which includes both destructive and intuitively helpful behaviors that nurses might incorporate in interactions with clients concerning sexual health. This level includes the nurses' internalized taboos, myths, and stereotypic responses toward sexual function and structure.

To be therapeutic, however, nurses must gain personal awareness of their feelings about sex and sexuality, requiring a move to the second or *basic* level. Awareness is seen as the key to this level and requires that nurses clarify their own values before attempting to assist clients. According to Mims and Swenson (1980), awareness is obtained through unbiased reading; objective evaluation of experiences, feedback, and group interactions; and introspection and self-assessment. At this basic level, nurses become able to raise their own consciousness. This is seen as the first step toward being qualified for intervention in the realm of human sexuality. To counsel pregnant clients, then, nurses would have to deal with personal feelings and biases concerning sex during pregnancy.

The third or *intermediate* level includes the communication skills of giving permission and giving information. The skills needed by the nurse at this level include the nursing process, communication, counseling, and teaching skills. Much effective intervention is channeled through the behaviors of information and permission giving. For example, during pregnancy, many couples ask about alternate means of pleasuring. They might want information concerning these alternative modes, such as masturbation, but they also may need permission to engage in such activities. Other common questions requiring information and permission giving involve sexual positioning, when and if intercourse should be suspended, and the effects of intercourse on the fetus.

The highest level in this model is the *advanced* level. It requires post baccalaureate preparation for the nurse to incorporate its interventions. These interventions include suggestion giving, therapy, educational programs, and research projects. An example of a sexual problem in the pregnant family that might require this level of intervention might be the husband who must engage in extramarital affairs while his wife is pregnant. Such patterns are likely to be too complex for the nurse who is not a specialist in this area. The appropriate level of intervention for the nonspecialist nurse is generally the intermediate level.

The Nursing Process in the Sexual Health of the Pregnant Family

The first phase is, of course, the assessment phase, the tool for which is the sexual history which can be found in a number of books dealing with human sexuality and nursing, such as Mims and Swenson (1980) or Woods (1984). A true picture of sexual structure and function cannot be obtained unless both the woman and her mate are present. Included in the assessment and sexual history during pregnancy will be information regarding (1) the clients' prepregnant sexual attitudes, behaviors, feelings, and beliefs; (2) medical diagnoses and findings concerned with the pregnancy, including due date, last menstrual period, and menstrual and other relevant history related to reproduction; (3) information from physical examinations and laboratory findings and other pertinent data from prenatal visits; (4) mental and emotional status and function, especially as it relates to the pregnancy; (5) perception of sex role, body image, and prepregnant family dynamics; and (6) family, social, and cultural data.

The second phase of the nursing process is the establishment of a nursing diagnosis related to sexuality and sexual function in the pregnant family or couple. Mims and Swenson's (1980) definition of appropriate goals for general nursing interventions gives direction as well for intervention with the pregnant family. Included are helping the pregnant couple (1) to acquire accurate knowledge in order to eliminate myths and misconceptions concerning sex and sex-role functon during pregnancy; (2) to determine and acknowledge their feelings concerned with sex during pregnancy and sex roles; (3) to explore various options, both for sexual behaviors during pregnancy and for patterns of role behaviors (that is, androgyny); (4) to achieve a mode for sexual gratification and improved function of roles during pregnancy; (5) to perceive similarities and differences in their own and their mate's sexual function and masculine/feminine role behaviors.

Intervention will include the nursing behaviors of information and permission giving. By and large, sexual intercourse is safe for the couple and may be encouraged during pregnancy.The couple may simply need permission to behave sexually during this period. Information may be given to the couple concerning the previously discussed physiological and psychological changes during the trimesters of pregnancy and their possible effects on desire and sexual function. Other areas of information or permission giving may concern different positions that may be adopted as the woman's abdomen enlarges, and different modes of pleasuring. These may include cunnilingus, as long as the man is cautioned not to blow into his mate's vagina. This practice has been shown to produce fatal air embolism in the woman due to entry of air into the placental circulation (Falleh, Leach, & Wilkinson, 1973).

According to Mims and Swenson (1980) penile-vaginal intercourse may be encouraged by the nurse except in the following situations:

1. Where there is a history of early miscarriage.
2. When the woman has uterine fibroids, uterine abnormalities, or

cervical incompetence. If cervical banding is done to tighten the cervix, intercourse can be resumed.

3. Where there is evidence of premature rupture of the amniotic membrane.
4. Where there is unexplained vaginal bleeding.
5. If there is abdominal pain.
6. Where there is a history of premature labor, in which case the couple should be cautioned to avoid orgasm, either through manual manipulation or intercourse. However, to date, there has been no conclusive link established between uterine spasm and initation of premature labor (Calhoun, et al., 1981).

Another area of information and permission giving that may be explored concerns sex-role function. The couple may be given "permission" to discuss feelings and preference concerning their relative masculine or feminine roles and how they would like to function during pregnancy and parenting. Information may be shared concerning modes of establishing more role flexibility, in an androgynous pattern of interactions. For example, the woman may need permission to lapse into a feminine-sex role pattern of dependency, without feeling guilt; or the man may need permission to make plans to nurture his infant-to-be, or to express his own "couvade" behaviors. All these areas need to be considered when assisting the pregnant family to attain a high level of sexual health and function during pregnancy.

SUMMARY

Sexual behavior is extremely complex, having structural and functional components on both an individual and family systems level. Further, it affects all spheres of life. Pregnancy is a time of disorganization and crisis for many families. Inherent patterns of sexuality in the individual and family system will determine the sexual well-being of the family during pregnancy. Nurses and other health care professionals, in order to deliver holistic care, may intervene to assist the couple in both determining sexual behaviors during pregnancy and also in restructuring sexual dynamics within the family system.

REFERENCES

Battacchi, M. (1978). Personality and stress factors in women's sexuality in pregnancy. In L. Carenzo, P. Pancher & L. Zichella (Eds)., *Clinical psychoneuroendocrinology in reproduction.* New York: Academic Press.

Baumrind, D. (1982). Are androgynous individuals more effective persons and parents? *Child Development, 53*(1), 44–75.

Bem, S.L. (1974). The measurement of psychological androgyny. *Journal of Consulting and Clinical Psychology, 42,* 155–62.

Bem, S. L. (1975). Sex role adaptability: One consequence of psychological androgyny. *Journal of Personality and Social Psychology, 31,* 634–663.

Bem, S.L., & Lenny, E. (1976). Sex typing and the avoidance of cross-sex behavior. *Journal of Personality and Social Psychology, 33,* 48–54.

Bemporad, J. (1980). *Child development in normality and psychopathology.* New York: Brunner/Mazel.

Bessoff, E., & Glass, G. (1982). The relationship between sex role and mental health: A meta-analysis of 26 studies. *Counseling Psychology, 10*(4), 105–112.

Calhoun, L., Selby, J., & King, E. (1981). The influence of pregnancy on sexuality: A review of current evidence. *Journal of Sex Research, 17*(2), 139–151.

Caplan, G. (1959). *Concepts of mental health and consultation.* Washington, DC: U.S. Department of Health, Education and Welfare.

Dameron, G.W. (1983). Helping couples cope with sexual changes pregnancy brings. *Contemporary Obstetrics and Gynecology, 21,* 23–37.

Falicov, C.V. (1973). Sexual adjustment during first pregnancy and postpartum. *American Journal of Obstetrics and Gynecology, 117,* 991–1000.

Falleh, A., Leach, W., & Wilkinson, C. (1973). Fatal air embolism in pregnancy resulting from orogenital sex play. *Forensic Science, 2,* 247–250.

Feldman, L.B. (1982). Sex roles and family dynamics. In F. Walsh (Ed), *Normal family processes.* New York: Guilford Press.

Feldman, S., & Aschenbrenner, B. (1983). Impact of parenthood on various aspects of masculinity and femininity: A short term longitudinal study. *Developmental Psychology, 19* (2), 1278–1289.

Hatfield, E., Greenberger, D., Traupmann, J., & Lambert, P. (1982). Equity and sexual satisfaction in recently married couples. *Journal of Sex Research, 18*(1), 18–32.

Katchadourian, H., & Lunde, D.T. (1972). *Fundamentals of human sexuality.* New York: Holt, Rinehart, and Winston.

Kenny, J. A. (1973). Sexuality of pregnant and breastfeeding women. *Archives of Sexual Behavior, 2,* 215–219.

Lenz, E., Soeken, K., Rankin, E., & Fishmen, S. (1985). Sex-role attributes, gender, and post-partal perceptions of the marital relationship. *Advances in Nursing Science, 7*(3), 49–60.

Lumley, J. (1978). Sexual feelings in pregnancy and after childbirth. *Australian and New Zealand Journal of Obstetrics and Gynecology, 18,* 114–117.

Masters, W., & Johnson, V. (1966). *Human sexual response.* Boston: Little, Brown.

Mims, F., & Swenson, M. (1980) *Sexuality: A nursing perspective.* New York: McGraw-Hill.

Nass, G., Libby, R., & Fisher, M. (1983). *Sexual choices.* Monterey CA: Wadsworth.

Nye, F.I. (1976). *Role structure and analysis of the family.* Beverly Hills, CA: Sage.

Osofsky, H. (1982). Expectant and new fatherhood as a developmental crisis. *Bulletin of Menninger Clinic, 46*(3), 209–230.

Osofsky, H., & Osofsky, J. (1980). *Answers for new parents: Adjusting to your role.* New York: Walker.

Osofsky, J., & Windle, M. (1978). Sex-role orientation, behavioral adaptability, and personal adjustment. *Sex Roles, 4,* 801–811.

Robson, K., Brant, H., & Kumar, R. (1981). Maternal sexuality during first pregnancy and after childbirth. *British Journal of Obstetrics and Gynecology, 88,* 882–889.

Safir, M.P. (1982). Psychological androgyny and sexual adequacy. *Journal of Sex and Marital Therapy, 8*(3), 228–240.

Selby, J., & Calhoun, L. (1981). Sexuality during pregnancy. In Ahmed, P. (Ed) *Pregnancy, childbirth, and parenthood.* New York: Elsevier North-Holland.

Stream, H. S. (1983). *The sexual dimension: A guide for the helping professional.* New York: Free Press.

Tolor, A., & DiGranzia, P. (1976). Sexual attitudes and behavior patterns during the following pregnancy. *Archives of Sexual Behavior, 5,* 539–551.

White, S., & Reamy, K. (1982). Sexuality and pregnancy: A review. *Archives of Sexual Behavior, 11*(5), 429–444.

Whitney, B. (1983). Sex role orientation and self-esteem: A critical meta-analytic review. *Journal of Personality and Social Psychology, 44*(4), 765–778.

Wiggins, J., & Holzmuller, A. (1981). Further evidence on androgyny and inter-personal flexibility. *Journal of Research in Personality, 15*(1), 67–80.

Woods, N. F., & Dery, G. K. (1984). Sexuality during pregnancy and lactation. In N. F. Woods (Ed.), *Human sexuality in health and illness.* St. Louis: C. V. Mosby.

Zuengler, K., & Neubeck, G. (1983). Sexuality: Developing togetherness. In H. McCubbin, & C. Figley (Eds.), *Stress and the family.* New York: Brunner/Mazel.

Chapter 5

Maternal Role Attainment

Few theorists today believe that evolving into the role of mother, at least in human beings, is an inevitable, instinctive event initiated by the biological act of giving birth to an infant. Giving birth does not guarantee that a woman can or wants to assume a mothering role to that infant, nor does it guarantee that she will be able to perform the tasks necessary to insure survival of the infant, or even that she will love her offspring. Assumption of the role of mother has been found to be similar to assumption of any other role relevant to society. It is seen as an active process requiring motivation on the part of the individual hoping to assume that role. Further, the role of mother is attained over a long period of time, not just when the infant appears in the external world. The roots of the maternal role are developed in a girl's childhood. During the pregnancy, a woman actively and progressively "works" on her role, desiring to assume the role behaviors of the "ideal" mother. Finally, after the birth of the infant and through interaction with the infant, the mother becomes bound-in to the maternal role.

THE PROCESS OF ROLE ATTAINMENT: AN OVERVIEW

To understand the specific processes inherent in assumption of the maternal role, a brief review of the process of role assumption in general is necessary. First, a role is social in nature, that is, it is defined by individuals in a particular society. Second, a role is manifest by behaviors and actions used in social situations or in interactions with others. A role, then, is defined as a set of expectations impinging on the occupant of a social position. These expectations are derived from society, from others who occupy the same role, and from one's self-expectations regarding the behaviors, attitudes, knowledge, values, and skills one should possess when occupying that role (Thornton & Nardi, 1975). This definition will be seen to be most relevant in understanding the process a woman undertakes when she assumes the maternal role. The term *role* is also defined by inherent behaviors; that is, it is a patterned sequence of learned actions performed by persons in interactions with others (Sarbin, 1954); it is further a group of specified behaviors demanded of or forbidden to the person who is in the role (Rosenberg, 1976). The prospective mother, to be truly in the role of mother, must learn role-appropriate skills and behaviors necessary for interacting successfully with a totally dependent, nonverbal infant. She also must learn what behaviors society prohibits to individuals mothering an infant.

How does a woman go about learning how to fit into the role of mother? In general, the decision to attain a role, plus the ability to adapt to it successfully, are determined by inherent (genetic) endowments and by interactions with the environment. Early in a girl's childhood, expectations that others, especially her parents, hold for the child herself help pattern the way she will become a mother and her expectations of herself in that role. Further, the society and culture in which the girl lives will also set forth parameters for role behaviors as a mother. Those who attempt to take their places within the role are greatly influenced by how they perceive that others, especially others in the same role, evaluate their role performance (Rosenberg, 1976). It is no mystery why the woman's most important role model as she moves into the maternal role is her own mother!

Anyone, including a prospective mother, who intends to assume a role engages in a specific process of acquisition. Thornton and Nardi (1975) describe a developmental stage approach consistent with the belief expressed here that assumption of the role of mother requires movement through progressive stages. For them, the stages of role assumption include

1. *Anticipatory phase.* Acquired role expectations are often incomplete, stereotypical, and unrealistic. "Shoulds" and "oughts" are stressed,

and appraisal of role functions tends to be unrealistic. In this stage, actual adaptation of the individual to the role may be impeded.

2. *Formal phase.* Newly in the role, the individual is made aware of explicit rules for role behavior and tends to follow these prescriptions rigidly rather than adjust them to personal needs. Little flexibility and variation in role performance are allowed at this phase.

3. *Informal phase.* The role taker learns unofficial, informal role expectations through interactions with others. Behaviors now begin to become more flexible, and alternative patterns of behavior for role performance become evident.

4. *Personal phase.* The role taker now has made the role his or her "own"—it is part of the self. One's own perceptions and modifications of behaviors and expectations of the role are formed. Satisfaction in the role is obtained if personal role modifications occur in a way that also meets personal needs. Role structure now enables the role taker to formulate and attain realistic goals desirable in the particular role.

FACTORS THAT AFFECT ROLE-TAKING BEHAVIORS

Rubin (1967, 1984) and others, such as Lederman (1984), who have done detailed qualitative data collection and analysis specifically on mothers, present some modifications of this basic process, which will be discussed in some depth later in this chapter. Other questions of importance to be considered concern factors that might affect role taking and role behaviors of the mother and her interactions with her infant. The literature reveals several variables that may affect role behavior and perhaps the ability to take on a role.

In one study, Richardson (1981) identifies work roles as important mediators of how parenting roles are manifest in behaviors. This relationship is further mediated by gender identity, race, and classification. In a study looking at relationships among employment status, role conflict, marital satisfaction, employment role attitude, and ease of transition to the maternal role, Majewski (1985) found no significant differences between employed and unemployed mothers in relation to role conflict. Mothers who perceived they had "careers," however, experienced more role conflict between worker, self, and spouse roles than did mothers who perceived they had "jobs."

Mothers experiencing role conflict had the most difficulty in making a transition to the maternal role, regardless of employment status. Marital satisfaction facilitated maternal role transition. When one considers the common social phenomenon of working and career-minded individuals seeking to become mothers, such variables become major issues in understanding the maternal role a woman assumes.

Another important variable discussed by Erikson (1960) and verified by later research is sense of identity within a role. Erikson describes the process of identity formation as being comprised of the individual's concern with her or his role, that is, how she or he appears to others. Another component is how she or he perceives the self in the role. Although Erikson speaks of identity formation as a specific task of adolescence, identity formation is seen as neither beginning nor ending with adolescence. It continues throughout life as one assumes new phase-appropriate roles, such as "mother." New mothers must reestablish a different sense of identity within the maternal role, and to do so they must redefine their sense of "self." The manner in which identity is established has great implications for the manner in which role behaviors are performed. Burke and Reitzes (1981), in a study of 640 college students, were able to demonstrate that identity will motivate behaviors that have meaning consistent with that identity. Thus, the sense of identity a mother has in the role will help determine her performance of mothering behaviors.

Culture is an all-pervasive variable that will affect maternal role taking. After an extensive review of research and literature on culture and childbearing, Aamodt (1978) concludes that culturally relevant content, related to the process of childbearing touches almost every aspect of social life in a culture. The cultural orientation of a community will allow that group to answer many socially vital questions: What processes distinguish a biological parent from a sociological parent? What appropriate rituals must accompany birth? What values are held with respect to roles of children, mother, father, and grandparent? What constitutes appropriate parenting and a "family unit"? What beliefs do individuals hold concerning the processes of conception, childbirth, and birth control?

It is not within the scope of this chapter to describe the manner in which a variety of cultures resolve these issues related to childbearing. The reader is referred to Clark's *Culture, Childbearing, Health Professionals*

(1978), which provides extensive descriptions of a variety of cultural groups' approaches to childbearing.

Finally, Sommers (1981) found that affective state (emotional range) possessed by an individual had an effect on role-taking behavior and role performance in a sample of female college students. This is an important consideration in a woman's assumption of the maternal role. At a time when emotional lability is common and affective state is not stable, role taking and performance in the role may be far more difficult to achieve.

THE PROCESS OF MATERNAL ROLE TAKING

Thus far, we have considered similarities between the process of assumption of the maternal role and role assumption in general. How is assumption of the maternal role unique? Certainly there is a definite physiological component (that is, the biological pregnancy and presence of the fetus) that is present throughout the process of maternal role assumption. There are also other differences.

As mentioned, the roots for evolving a role of mother are found in childhood. The model the girl has that will be highly instrumental in shaping perceptions of not only gender role but also maternal role is, of course, her own mother. This process begins early and continues through various developmental stages. Girls have been found to be more dependent on parental evaluations and parental self-concept for development of their roles than are boys (Gecas, Calonico, & Darwin, 1974). Thus, a girl may well be exceedingly aware of and sensitive to her mother's (and to an extent, her father's) attitudes and actions concerning the maternal role and its associated behaviors. Throughout a girl's life in the family of origin, she is encouraged to continue to identify with her mother (Hoffman, 1975).

Studying a somewhat different time frame, Mercer (1985) examined the process of maternal role attainment in three age groups (15 to 19 years, 20 to 29 years, and 30 to 42 years) over the first year of motherhood. She found that role attainment in all three groups—indicated by feelings of love for the infant, gratification in the maternal role, observed maternal behaviors, and handling an irritated infant—did not demonstrate a positive linear increase over the year. Rather, these indicators peaked at 4 months after delivery and then declined at 8 months. Data from interviews indicated that complex infant developmental behaviors at 8 to 12 months produced feelings of incompetence in these mothers. Thus, the process does not end with birth; nor does the process go in an entirely predictable upward pattern. Maternal role attainment has its peaks and low points, even after the infant is on the scene.

For purposes of this book, however, the focus of maternal role attainment and development is the phase of pregnancy. Two major investigators and theoreticians are particularly prominent in this area and will be discussed in some depth. These are Reva Rubin and Regina Lederman.

RUBIN'S CONCEPTUAL FRAMEWORK FOR MATERNAL ROLE ASSUMPTION

Reva Rubin has been and remains one of the foremost theoreticians concerning the psychosocial aspects of mothering. Rubin originally developed a framework for the process of maternal role assumption in 1967 (Rubin, 1967). In a new publication (Rubin, 1984), she has revised some of her conceptualizations of the process. Both the old and new framework will be discussed here, since most nurses are familiar with the earlier formulations.

Rubin (1984) sees movement into a maternal role as a process that occurs not only with the first pregnancy but also with each successive pregnancy. It is an active, volitional process where the woman moves closer to her "ideal" in terms of desired attributes and performance as a mother. "The outcome is more than a sentimental attachment and more than a role that is stepped into and out of again. There is a belonging as a part of the whole personality, bound-in and inseparable, a maternal identity" (p. 38).

The development of the maternal role (or, as Rubin (1984) describes it, a maternal identity for this child) is effected in a progressive series of cognitive operations manifest in conceptual and behavioral modes that parallel the development of the pregnancy and growth of the fetus. Further, the maternal role is intimately linked to achievement of certain "maternal tasks." "It is the involvement in the continuous and increasingly more complex maternal tasks, with the commitment for effectiveness in these tasks, that makes for the binding-in to the maternal identity in relation to this child" (Rubin, 1984, p. 54). Again, the tasks are self-imposed and motivated by the desire to have *this* child and be competent as a mother to it. Both the cognitive operations of maternal role attainment and the tasks that must be accomplished to bind-in the maternal role or identity will be discussed.

Cognitive Operations

Rubin (1967) originally formulated a framework for maternal role assumption involving four cognitive operations: mimicry/role play, fantasy, introjection/projection/rejection, and grief work. These original operations have been reformulated into three operations: replication, fantasy, and dedifferentiation (Rubin, 1984).

Replication. This cognitive operation is seen by Rubin (1984) as the volitional search for and trying on of separate valued elements in behavior and attitude which are esteemed by society. This constitutes the primary mode of incorporation or "binding-in" of the maternal role. Replication is self-initiated; the woman actively searches out new desired elements of the maternal role to be replicated or taken on by the self. In this early phase, most replicative behavior is not taken in or integrated into the personality but serves as a bridge or an intent to bind-in attitudes and behaviors of subsequent operations.

Mimicry/role play, elements of Rubin's (1967) old schema, are seen as the two forms of replicative behaviors. Mimicry is the first suboperation and constitutes literal "copying" of the practice and customs of other women in the same situation, or of women who have successfully achieved these situations, especially the woman's own mother. Also copied are recommendations of "experts"—health care professionals who interact with the woman. Mimicry eventually becomes more sophisticated. The woman continues to sample attitudes and behaviors and gains some knowledge of which are the desired or undesired ones.

The second form of replication, role play, is a trying-on of the maternal role. Instead of just modeling behaviors, the pregnant woman now selects a partner, usually an infant or child from her immediate environment, with whom to practice role behaviors. Feedback from the role partner is closely observed by the woman for signs of positive or negative response to mothering behaviors. If the partner responds in a positive manner, the woman's confidence in her evolving role of mother is increased. However, if her maternal role behavior is rejected by the partner, there will be a loss of confidence in herself as a potentially competent mother. While role playing is seen more frequently in primiparas, multiparas role play with their husbands and children "as if" the new baby were born and present.

Rubin (1984) summarizes the cognitive operation of replication in mimicry and role plays as "a bridge to becoming a mother, . . . volitional acts, . . . a preliminary binding-in to a maternal identity (p. 39).

Fantasy. Fantasy state during pregnancy as a specific psychosocial entity on its own will be discussed in Chapter 6. Here, Rubin (1984) discusses fantasy as an intrinsic component of maternal role-taking (Lederman (1984) sees fantasy in this light as well). Thus, the discussion here will be limited to the role of fantasy as a cognitive operation in assumption of the maternal role or identity.

Rubin sees the process of role assumption moving inside the woman via the transactions of fantasy. Fantasy is defined as the projection into the future, in imagery, of the mother and her child-to-be. Stimulus for fantasy is said to originate in models and situations of replication. In fantasy, however, there is no third person; there is just the mother and her fantasy child. In fantasy, the mother can cognitively explore a variety of situations and experiences she will find herself in with her future infant. This operation is seen as a vital one for binding-in to the child-to-be and to the self as mother.

The nature of the fantasies changes throughout the pregnancy, ranging from, in the first two trimesters, idyllic daydreams of the baby (including gender, behavior, and looks) and of nurturing the baby, to fearful daydreams concerned with the child, self, and the impending labor and delivery in the third trimester.

In Rubin's (1984) new conceptualization, grief work is incorporated into the cognitive operation of fantasy. As the woman binds in, in fantasy, to her future life with the baby, there is a loosening and realigning of affiliative bonds to other persons. There is also a loosening of parts of her own personality, aspirations, activities, lifestyle, and life space in the world. At first there is resistance to giving up these facets of life, but as the mother-to-be binds in to the child in fantasies and to her role in mothering this child, she is able to disengage and distance herself from other roles, commitments, aspirations, and involvements. Part of this function of fantasy in resolving grief involves review in memory of past stages of life no longer compatable with the evolving future with a child. This review in disengagement from bonds of a former identity at times requires a listener and at times must be done silently in thought, alone (Rubin, 1984).

Thus, through fantasies of the future that allow the mother to bind in to her child-to-be and her new role, and through fantasy review of the past that allows grief work to release her from past roles, the mother-to-be moves one step closer to making the maternal role her own.

Dedifferentiation. This cognitive operation constitutes the final phase in maternal role assumption in the current scheme and incorporates the former scheme's operation of introjection/projection/rejection. In reaching this last operation, past operations have greatly changed the woman. Accommodations made in the wish for replication, felt experiences in fantasy, and preparatory relinquishment and reorganization of bonds to self and to others now form a substantive core of maternal identity. With this core, the woman is still receptive to elements for replicability of the ideal. Now, however, there is no longer a taking on in mimicry. Instead, the operation available to the mother, as described by Rubin (1984), is dedifferentiation. This cognitive operation is said to be an examination and evaluation of the attitudes and behaviors of a model for goodness of fit with the current self-image as mother. There is a trying-on, an introjection of a newly modeled element, then a projection of the mental image of the self with that new element in action or in appearance, and the decision to accept or to reject the new element as a congruent part of the self.

The complete attainment of the maternal role or identity, although much of the process has occurred in pregnancy, awaits birth of the infant and an identification of the child in reality. "The dedifferentiation of self from models, without closure to further replicable ideal attributes, immediately precedes the establishment of the maternal identity" (Rubin, 1984, p. 51). Rubin makes one final point concerning formation of the maternal role or identity, which is that attachment to the child-to-be and formation of a maternal role and identity are interdependent parts of the same process. Without the desire for the child, there is no active motivation to assume the maternal role.

Maternal Tasks

To attain the maternal role, the mother must accomplish certain self-imposed and increasingly complex tasks during pregnancy. The tasks, which number four, are addressed by means of the taking-on, taking-in, and letting go operations of replication, fantasy (with disengagement), and dedifferentiation. "With supportive inputs from family and other significant persons on the one hand, and with encouraging feedback from this child (to-be) on the other hand, the fabric of a maternal identity is actively woven in themes of the maternal tasks" (Rubin, 1984, p. 54). The four maternal tasks, according to Rubin, are safe passage, acceptance by others, binding-in to the child, and giving of oneself.

Safe Passage. To accomplish this task, the mother must seek and ensure safe passage for her fetus and herself through the course of pregnancy and childbirth. While in the first trimester, the focus of "being safe" is on herself; by the third trimester, the pregnant woman sees herself and her fetus as inseparable, so what constitutes danger for one is danger for the other. Thus, labor and delivery are seen as "double jeopardy" to self and child. Ensurance of safe passage is done primarily by acquiring knowledge of what to expect and of how to cope with and control phenomena and events during pregnancy and childbirth.

Acceptance by Others. Childbearing stresses the social fabric of a woman's established relationships in the primary social group of the family. Much of the stress of moving into the maternal role will be mediated by the quality of relationships within the family, and the manner in which family members, especially the prospective father, accept the pregnancy, the infant-to-be, and the life changes that will be necessary to incorporate the infant into the family group. Acceptance of the coming child requires an awareness of certain personal sacrifices and a willingness to let go of some aspects of the former life. What is most important, according to Rubin (1984), is acceptance by each member of the family of these sacrifices made by self and other members. Acceptance must also be achieved by other children in the family, who must come to accept certain deprivations and delayed gratifications inherent in the enlarging family.

Binding-in to the Child. To attain maternal identity, the prospective mother must achieve the task of establishing a form of direct communication or experience between herself and the fetus. Only in this way is the infant-to-be transformed from a remote "theoretical model" to personhood, an individual self that gives purpose and significance to becoming the mother of *this* child. In general, fetal movements begin to transform the "theoretical" child to a real, living child for the mother-to-be. The awareness of the "real" child, not just a pregnancy, adds a new dimension of affectional bonds and reciprocal relatedness to the woman's experience. Such bonds, established with the fetus during pregnancy, are the roots of the maternal-infant relationship after birth.

Giving of Oneself. This is seen by Rubin (1984) as the most intricate and complex task of childbearing and childbirth. The woman has progressive demands and deprivations placed on her body self, as well as her psychological and social self, throughout the pregnancy. She must come to see that these demands have a purpose and, in essence, are an important form of giving of herself to the unborn child. As the demands imposed by pregnancy are mastered, the woman works at the essential and substantive meaning of giving to the infant-to-be. In order to "give" herself to the child, the mother must be "given to" by others, especially her family members, but also the professionals who care for her.

LEDERMAN'S CONCEPTUAL FRAMEWORK FOR MATERNAL ROLE ASSUMPTION

Rubin's (1967, 1984) formulations provide an observable sequence of stages, steps, and operations a woman must pass through to attain the maternal role. Other investigators have also studied the process by which one moves into the role of being a mother to an infant. One empirical study that added information concerned with maternal role assumption was done by Lederman and her associates (Lederman, Lederman, Work, & McAnn, 1979). Lederman (1984) sees maternal role assumption or, as she describes it, "identification with a motherhood role," as part of the larger process of psychosocial development in pregnancy.

Lederman's work evolved from a research project that investigated the relationship of maternal psychosocial adaptation in pregnancy to maternal anxiety and labor progress during childbirth (Lederman et al., 1979). From analysis of data, seven personality dimensions or "areas of developmental challenge" were defined, one of them being identification with a motherhood role.[1] Although Lederman's first study looked only at primigravidas, it gives much insight into factors that contribute to assumption of the maternal role.

Lederman describes (1984) the goal of identification with a motherhood role as taking the developmental step of being a woman-without-child to being a woman-with-child. They indicate that it can be thought of as a process characterized by progressive emphasis in the mother's thinking away from the single self and toward the mother-baby unit. Identification of the motherhood role involves two important factors: how motivated the woman is to assume that role and the extent to which the woman has prepared for a motherhood role. Further, identification of the role is closely related to the woman's relationship with her own mother. These three areas will be discussed in this section. In Lederman et al.'s, research, anxiety or conflict concerning the motherhood role is associated with fears about labor that relate to helplessness, pain, loss of control, and loss of self-esteem. Further, difficulty in identifying a motherhood role is associated with slower progress in labor.

Motivation for Motherhood

This factor includes concepts of how much a woman wants to become a mother, especially her interest in and ability to nurture and empathize with a child. In addition, motivation for motherhood includes the woman's perception of motherhood as fulfilling or as being an important event in her life. Motivation is questioned if a woman's thoughts about a child are infrequent, aversive, avoided, or denied; or if the woman seems to desire the pregnancy and not the child (Lederman, 1984).

Preparation for Motherhood

Based on her research findings, Lederman (1984) asserts that it is not sufficient for a woman just to want to be a mother. She also needs to prepare for her new role by envisioning herself as a mother and con-

---

[1]Although identification is discussed as a separate dimension here, users of the Lederman Prenatal Self-Evaluation Questionnaire for purpose of maternal development assessment can use the instrument only in its complete form, with all seven dimensional scales.

templating her life as a woman with a child. The main way this happens, according to Lederman, is through fantasy and dreaming (including daydreams and night dreams). In this study, fantasy and dreams, both day and night, were not sharply differentiated. Preparation also includes a woman's life experiences, particularly the availability of a role model; the degree of conflict resolution a woman attains; and the need to attach to the baby.

Fantasy and Dreams. Fantasy is made up of three processes: envisioning oneself as a mother, thinking about characteristics one would like to have as a mother, and anticipating future life changes that will be necessary with a child. Blocks to these processes are seen as excessive doubts and fears that can interfere with fantasy, an inability to project life change and find compensation in the infant-to-be, and an inability to engage in abstract thought or fantasy (Lederman, 1984).

Dreaming is important in identifying the motherhood role, as dream content tends to parallel a woman's actual concerns in waking life. Further, emotional content often is vivid, indicating dreams (night dreams) are important to the woman. Lederman (1984) identified five categories of dreams: reliving childhood, school dreams, motherhood-career conflict dreams, confidence-in-maternal-skills dreams, and food and infant intactness dreams.

Lederman (1984) summarizes the importance of fantasy and dreams in allowing the woman to identify with the motherhood role: "The content of dreams often presents a mixture of past experiences and present perceived tasks. . . . Fantasy and dreaming help her (the gravida) prepare for what is ahead. In this way, the trials of childbirth and the skills of mothering are rehearsed" (p. 54).

Life Experience. Lederman (1984) found that a woman's ability to fantasize depended on her life experiences, especially how she was nurtured. If the woman was well nurtured, she generally had a good role model for mothering to emulate. Further, positive experience and the ability to identify with other women were seen as positive factors in assuming the role of mother.

Conflict Resolution. Every woman in Lederman's (1984) study was seen to bring some conflicts to the pregnancy. However, if a woman's doubts were not overwhelming, conflicts were worked out over the course of the pregnancy, allowing the woman to reach an appropriate level of preparedness and confidence. A major conflict reported by some of Lederman's sample was over the desire both to be a mother and to identify oneself as a career woman. If one desire or the other was amenable to adjustment, the conflict could be resolved. However, sustained motherhood-career conflicts, due to the gravida's unwillingness to let go of parts of her career role or due to perception of the motherhood role as unrewarding, were seen to raise feelings of inadequacy regarding mothering.

Maternal Attachment Behavior. This factor was associated with future acceptance, nurturance, and protection of the child and was seen as a process that began well before the birth of the infant. Attachment behavior includes recognition of the individuality and attributes of the fetus-child, imaginative role rehearsal, thoughts about giving oneself to the child, and fantasy about interacting with the child. Behaviors associated with attachment, as identified by Lederman's (1984) subjects, include selection of names, evaluation of feeding methods, talking to the fetus, and touching or stroking fetal parts. The development of attachment to the fetus (and child-to-be) can be seen as a transition during which the mother gains a sense of the child. This transition is associated with increased feelings of maternal competency and effectiveness and thus greatly affects identification with motherhood role.

Woman's Relationship with Her Own Mother

Lederman's (1984) and Lederman et al.'s (1979) studies clearly identify relationship with the mother as a factor in a woman's identification with a motherhood role. The gravida's relationship with her mother is one of the important dimensions in psychosocial adjustment during pregnancy.

Four components are important in the gravida's relationship with the grandmother (her mother): (1) availability of the grandmother to the woman, in the past and during pregnancy; (2) the grandmother's reaction to the pregnancy, especially her acceptance of the grandchild-to-be and her acknowledgment of her daughter as a mother; (3) the grandmother's respect for her daughter's autonomy, as demonstrated by relating to the gravida as a mature adult rather than a child; and (4) the grandmother's willingness to reminisce, with her daughter, about her own childbearing and childrearing experiences.

On the opposite side of the coin, Lederman et al. (1979) discerned that the daughter (the gravida) also contributes to the quality of the relationship to her mother (the grandmother). Her ability to empathize with her mother's experiences as a parent and with the changes her mother must go through in transition to her new role as grandparent are seen as important in the mother–daughter relationship.

Lederman (1984) indicates, in summary, that, if the gravida's mother is available to her and their relationship is a mutual one, the mother will be supportive to the woman during pregnancy and childbirth. This mother, then, will serve as a constructive role model for the gravida and can help her (the gravida) establish an identification with the motherhood role. In the study the gravida's identification of a motherhood role was facilitated by a good relationship with her mother and was associated with fewer fears related to labor and delivery. A poor relationship with the mother was found to be related to prolonged labor. Thus, Lederman et al.'s research and theoretical formulations tend to confirm the importance of the mother-grand-mother link during the phase of pregnancy and in the assumption of the maternal role.

COMPARISON OF THE TWO FRAMEWORKS

While Rubin's (1967,1984) and Lederman's (1984; Lederman et al., 1979) formulations evolved from different types of observations, occurred at different times, and used different names for concepts, there are great similarities in their theories concerned with how a woman moves into the maternal role. Some key themes are repeated in both formulations: the role of fantasy, the ability to resolve conflicts, the relationship of the woman to her mother, the importance of role models, and the ability to attach to the fetus. These two generally compatible although independent formulations give much support to the belief that there are certain inherent mechanisms in the process of becoming a mother. Absence or inability to pass through these elements may impede the process of assumption of the maternal role. Further, nursing interventions might be directed toward assisting the mother to incorporate the appropriate mechanisms or key factors into her process of role attainment.

ROLE CONFLICT AND ATTAINMENT
OF THE MATERNAL ROLE

Assumption of a role does not always proceed smoothly. For several reasons, a person may not "fit" into a particular role. Such situations are commonly labeled role conflicts and continually occur for individuals who must function in a complex social structure (Minkler & Biller, 1979). Role conflict may occur in several ways. For example, there may be major discrepancies between the anticipated role and the actual, experienced role. Large shifts from familiar to unfamiliar roles, or roles that have conflicting but desired goals, may also produce role conflict. Further, inadequate preparation for the role or vague and ambiguous role definitions may produce role conflict.

Another potential source of role conflict stems from an individual's membership in mutiple groups. It is likely that at least one role necessary for social interactions in one group will be incompatible with a role necessary for interactions in a second group. The necessity of giving up or altering one or both roles may produce conflict for the individual.

These general situations point to several potential situations that may directly produce conflict in a woman attempting to move into the maternal role.

Origins of Role Conflict during Pregnancy

Inability to Achieve the "Good" Mother Role. Role conflict will increase if the mother believes that she cannot imitate the "good mother" of her childhood or has unrealistic expectations of the behaviors she will perform as the "good mother." If perceptions of her own mother are unrealistic and idealistic, she may fear her inability, or be unable to emulate the desired behaviors. She then perceives that she functions in the role as the "bad mother" (Jessner, Weigert, & Foy, 1970).

Lack of Knowledge and Preparation for the Maternal Role. In his now classic work on parenting, LeMasters (1957) describes the lack of preparation that individuals in modern society have for assuming roles of mother and father. In a nuclear family, guidelines for parenting are ambiguous and role models less apparent. Stressors include the rapid necessity to redesign old roles and adapt to new ones; reassess goals, values, and priorities associated with new roles; and determine alternative means of gratification from the new roles. Other investigators have also pointed to the lack of guidelines for successful parenting and the abruptness of the transition to parenthood at the birth of the child (Rossi, 1968).

Although some of this source of conflict may be alleviated by the current trend toward childbirth preparation during pregnancy and by family living courses in high school, this problem in role assumption will probably continue as society becomes more complex and mobile and the role of parent becomes more and more ambiguous and unclear.

Career Conflicts. Lederman (1984) clearly identifies the maternal-role/career-role conflict in her discussion of maternal dreams during pregnancy. Women in her sample equated total loss of the career role as loss of self. Kutzner and Toussie-Weingarten (1984) identify three factors that prompt the woman with children to work outside the home or pursue a career: economic, societal (the blurring of traditional roles of mother and father, and emergence of androgynous roles), and personal. These personal factors include self-respect, self-confidence, and independence gained from a career (Lancaster, 1975). The crucial question, according to these authors, is whether or not a woman can successfully integrate career roles and family roles.

Conflicts in Disengaging from Past Life Roles. Rubin's (1984) discussion of the grief work that must occur as a woman gives up her previous life to accept a new life with an infant encompasses career conflicts but tends to broaden to the whole of the past life space and style. Binding-in to the fantasy child is said to promote loosening and distancing from other roles, all replete with their commitments, aspirations, and involvements. A key to giving up past roles is the acceptance of the new roles involved with the infant-to-be and the feeling that the child compensates for what is given up. If the woman does not perceive compenation as adequate, role conflict may occur.

Role-Conflict Resolution during Pregnancy

It is given that, in assuming the maternal role, some level of role conflict is likely to develop. What are the mechanisms used for resolving these conflicts? A useful formulation of this process comes from Hall (1972) who identifies three alternatives:

1. *Structural role redefinition.* This mechanism involves redefining one's expectations of appropriate role performance by oneself and others, by negotiating a new set of expectations for the role that everyone can agree upon. For example, a mother may desire to raise her children in an androgynous fashion. Her own mother may initially dis-

approve; however, upon discussion, both redefine the role of the mother in raising children into a gender identity.

2. *Personal role redefinition.* This mechanism involves a change in one's perceptions and attitudes toward one's role, rather than an alteration of one's expectations through negotiation. The individual resolving conflict in this manner would change the perception of the role without attempting a compromise with other roles. For example, the mother just described would give up her belief about a mother's role in rearing androgynous children and behave in a manner that others see as appropriate.

3. *Reactive role behavior.* The individual attempts to meet all real or imagined expectations concerning a role. Such an attempt to master role conflict (for example, between the maternal role and career role) would prompt the "superwoman" syndrome. In this situation, a woman feels she must be a perfect, ideal mother *and* a perfect, ideal career woman. Such expectations are highly unrealistic and will provide a poor resolution to the role-conflict.

Van deVliert (1981) also proposes a framework for role-conflict resolution. His thesis rests on the finding that, in most situations, only one of the conflicting roles is seen as legitimate, or as having the most positive sanctions attached to it, or both. In this case, an individual can resolve the conflict by choosing the most positive role over the other. When both conflicting roles are seen as legitimate or illegitimate and simultaneously associated or not associated with positive sanctions, the cognitive mechanisms of compromise and/or avoidance will be used to resolve the conflict. Thus, the mother who sees that both her maternal role and her career role are legitimate and have equal positive sanctions associated with them will negotiate a compromise allowing her to keep both roles in a modified form. However, if only the maternal role is seen as legitimate and also has the best sanctions attached to it, the mother may choose the maternal role and give up the career role.

The important key in role-conflict resolution is the role taker's perception of the conflicting roles. The nurse will need to consider perception of role when attempting to assist the prospective mother in resolving role conflicts.

NURSING ASSESSMENT FOR THE
MOTHER IN ROLE CONFLICT

As with physiological dysfunction, presence of role conflict, a psychological dysfunction, will present signs and symptoms. Assessment and diagnosis of physiological symptoms is not always simple and clear-cut. One symptom may indicate several different pathological conditions. This situation is certainly more extreme when the nurse must assess cognitive signs and symptoms and come to the nursing diagnosis of "role conflict in assumption of the maternal role." The literature, however, and especially Rubin's (1984) and Lederman's (1984) discussions of inherent factors and steps that should appear in role assumption, does give direction to the diagnosis of conflict with the maternal role. The following are some of the possible signs that can be assessed by the nurse working with the pregnant woman.

Lack of Role Models for Motherhood. The woman who is totally isolated from women during the course of her pregnancy may be at risk for developing role conflict due to lack of guidelines for maternal role behavior. It would be impossible to replicate maternal behaviors without any models present. This situation may be modified further by past experience with potential maternal role models.

Absence of or Alienation from the Mother or Mother Substitute. This clue is related to the first but assumes greater importance when one considers the demonstrated importance of the link during pregnancy between the pregnant woman and her own mother. The present and past availability (both physical and psychological) of the woman's mother will be instrumental in how harmoniously she moves into the maternal role.

Inability to Engage in Fantasy about the Infant-to-Be and Future Life with the Infant. While inability to fantasize is seen elsewhere as a symptom of other problems in becoming a mother (see Chapter 6), it is viewed here as one of the possible indicators of maternal role conflict. Fantasy is seen by both Rubin (1984) and Lederman (1984) as a primary mode of "practicing" the maternal role before the birth of the infant. It further assists with binding-in to the future infant, a parallel process to assumption of the maternal role.

Inability to Resolve Grief over Disengagement from Past Roles. If the pregnant woman cannot accept life with an infant as adequate compensation for past roles and role behaviors that must be given up or greatly modified with birth of the child, she is a prime candidate for role conflict.

Inability to Visualize Life Change Necessitated by Birth of an Infant. The woman who does not perceive that having an infant will change her current lifestyle at all may have great difficulty adapting to the maternal role.

Inability to Insure the Infant-to-Be of a Safe Birth. Safe passage is one of the tasks Rubin (1967, 1984) sees as necessary to attaining the maternal role. The current concern with high-risk pregnancy needs to incorporate the potential problem that the at-risk mother may have in insuring her future infant of a safe birth.

Presence or Absence of Support Systems. Rubin (1984) speaks of the acceptance of others as vital in moving into the maternal role. Gaining acceptance of significant others for the pregnancy and infant-to-be is a task of pregnancy not only for the woman to attain. Acceptance of maternal role behaviors by the partner is also necessary, to allow the mother to feel confident in the role. Significant others, particularly the infant's father, who reject the pregnancy, infant-to-be, and/or maternal behaviors, may well produce great role conflict in the pregnant woman.

Evidence of Rejection of the Fetus. Since development of affectional bonds parallels assumption of the maternal role and provides motivation for achieving maternal tasks, rejection of the fetus will jeopardize role assumption.

Poor Motivation for Motherhood. This is similar to the preceding item. If the woman lacks motivation to be a mother and does not desire a child, she is likely to experience much role conflict.

Lack of Preparation for Motherhood. If the mother completely ignores all aspects of preparation for the impending birth—that is, if she has not cognitively prepared for or thought about labor, delivery, and care of the infant, or made preparations for the infant (nesting behaviors)—this behavior may signal conflict in the role of mother.

Ability to Resolve Conflicts and Extent of Conflict Resolution. By the time of the birth, a woman should have given some thought to how she intends realistically to resolve her multiple conflicting roles. If plans for resolution are unrealistic, or the woman has not even made any attempts at resolution, role crisis is a probability.

NURSING INTERVENTIONS

Again, based on the literature and the preceding list of possible signs indicating role crisis in achieving the maternal role, potential interventions designed to help the gravida resolve crisis and move into the maternal role emerge.

Encourage Fantasy

Encourage the pregnant woman to fantasize about her infant-to-be and about nurturing the baby. The nurse can easily engage the pregnant woman in discussing plans for the future with her baby and thus foster the mother's imagination. Many mothers need to be given permission to daydream, because it is viewed by many in our mechanistic society as childish and a waste of time. Further, the nurse may encourage the woman to remember and discuss her night dreams.

Assist the Woman in Gaining Information

This intervention can be accomplished in several ways. If the woman lacks role models and has no access to her mother, groups may provide the necessary models. For women late in pregnancy, of course, there are childbirth preparation groups of various types. The mother can be encouraged to discuss plans for childcare, perception of life changes, and so on with other women in her situation, within the group itself. For those in earlier stages of pregnancy, groups may also serve to expose the woman to other pregnant women.

Helping the woman prepare cognitively by encouraging her to read about necessary skills for caring for an infant may help her feel more confident in her evolving role. Further, she may be encouraged to try out parenting skills, by babysitting or being around friend's children.

Finally, the female nurse may serve as a role model for mothering behaviors, in either a professional or personal sense, through discussing other pregnant women and their approaches during pregnancy, talking about child and infant care, and sharing her own personal pregnancy, childbirth, and childrearing experiences.

Encourage Communication and Support

At some level, the nurse must work with the entire family of the woman having a conflict in assuming the maternal role. Encouraging open communication and sharing of both positive and negative feelings may assist significant others in accepting the pregnancy, coming child, and potential life changes. When family members, especially the infant's father, accept the pregnancy, they can support the mother in her role-taking activities.

Help the Mother to Clarify the Problem

While the nurse cannot clarify a situation for the pregnant woman, she can serve as a sounding board to enable the woman to clarify her own perception of her role and why she is having conflicts in assuming it. For example, a mother-to-be might not be aware that she has not properly grieved her past life, which she knows she must relinquish with the birth of the child. Through interactions with the nurse, she may become aware that the unfinished grief has not allowed her to disengage from her past life and find compensation in the child-to-be. Thus, she may resent the future child and have difficulty in evolving into the mother of *this* child. When the situation is clarified, the gravida may then engage in appropriate reminiscing, to resolve her grief about her past life.

Support the Woman in Conflict-Resolution Activities

Again, the nurse cannot resolve the gravida's conflict for her; however, the nurse can help the woman use appropriate conflict-resolution processes. For example, the nurse can help the pregnant woman to assess her perceptions of the legitimacy of two conflicting goals, often times that of mother and that of career woman. She can assist the gravida to assess the positive and negative sanctions incorporated in each role and to decide upon the desired mode of resolution. In this instance, if the mother sees both roles as equally important to her, she may decide upon a realistic compromise in activities associated with both roles. This might mean finding childcare during the day but modifying her job to eliminate extensive and overnight travel.

Referral

Finally, it is incumbent upon the nurse to determine when she or he can no longer help the pregnant woman, through counseling or crisis-resolution techniques, and when more intensive professional assistance is required to assist the woman in resolving her maternal role conflicts. For example, a deep-seated and unresolvable ambivalence of the gravida toward her own mother may make it impossible, without much intense treatment, for her ever to mother a child adequately or to assume the maternal role. The nurse with a maternal-child specialty does not generally have the skills required to do in-depth therapy. At this point, the nurse would recognize her or his limitations and would refer the pregnant woman in conflict to a clinical nurse specialist in psychiatric mental health nursing, or to a psychologist, psychiatrist, or other appropriate professional.

SUMMARY

The process of maternal role assumption is by no means simple and automatic. The mother-to-be must actively wish for and work at achieving the maternal role. Although there are impediments to assumption of the maternal role, there also is much about the process that is natural. We have identified and discussed both kinds of factors. Thus, there are guidelines to follow in nursing interventions with the pregnant woman as she strives to achieve the maternal role.

REFERENCES

Aamodt, A. (1978). Culture. In A. Clark (Ed.), *Culture, childbearing, health professionals.* Philadelphia: F.A. Davis.

Burke, P., & Reitzes, C. (1981). The link between identity and role performance. *Social Psychology Quarterly, 4*(2), 83–92.

Clark, A. (Ed.). (1978). *Culture, childbearing, health professionals.* Philadelphia: F. A. Davis.

Erikson, E. (1960). Identity and identity diffusion. In C. Gordon & K. Gergen (Eds.), *The self in social interaction,* vol. 1, New York: John Wiley.

Gecas, V., Caloncio, J., & Darwin, T. (1974). The development of self-concept in the child: Mirror theory versus model theory. *The Journal of Social Psychology, 92,* 67–76.

Hall, D. (1972). A model of coping with role conflict: The role behavior of college educated women. *The Administrative Quarterly, 17,* 471–486.

Hoffman, W. (1975). Early childhood experiences and women's achievement motives. In M. Mednica, S. Tangri, & L. Hoffman, (Eds.). *Women and achievement: Social and motivational analysis.* New York: John Wiley.

Jessner, L., Weigert, E., & Foy, J. (1970).The development of parental attitudes in pregnancy. In E. J. Anthony & T. Benedek (Eds.), *Parenthood, its psychology and psychopathology.*Boston: Little, Brown.

Kutzner, S., & Toussie-Weingarten, C. (1984). Working parents: The dilemma of childrearing and career. *Topics in Clinical Nursing, 6*(3), 30–37.

Lancaster, J. (1975). Coping mechanisms for the working mother. *American Journal of Nursing, 75*(8), 1322–1323.

Lederman, R. (1984). *Psychosocial adaptation in pregnancy: assessment of seven dimensions of maternal development.* East Norwalk, CT: Appleton-Century-Crofts.

Lederman, R., Lederman, E., Work, B., & McAnn, D. (1979). Relationship of psychological factors in pregnancy to progress in labor. *Nursing Research 28,* 94–97.

LeMasters, E. (1957). Parenthood in crisis. *Marriage and Family Living, 7,* 352–355.

Majewski, J. (1985). Conflicts, satisfactions, and attitudes during transition to the maternal role. *Nursing Research, 35*(1), 10–14.

Mercer, R. (1985). The process of maternal role attainment over the first year. *Nursing Research, 34*(4), 198–204.

Minkler, M., & Biller, R. (1979). Role shock: A tool for conceptualizing stresses accompanying disruptive role transitions. *Human Relations, 32*(2), 125–140.

Richardson, M. (1981). Occupation and family roles: A neglected intersection. *Counseling Psychologist, 9*(4), 13–23.

Rosenberg, M. (1976). *Conceiving the self.* New York: Basic Books.

Rossi, A. (1968). Transition to parenthood. *Journal of Marriage and the Family, 30,* 26–39.

Rubin, R. (1967). Attainment of the maternal role. *Nursing Research, 16*(3), 237–246.

Rubin, R. (1984). *Maternal identity and the maternal experience.* New York: Springer.

Sarbin, T. (1954). Role theory. *Handbook of social psychology,* vol. 1. Cambridge, MA: Addison Wesley.

Sommers, S. (1981). Emotionally reconsidered: The role of cognition in emotional responsiveness. *Journal of Personality and Social Psychology, 41*(3), 553–561.

Thornton, R., & Nardi, P. (1975). The dynamics of role acquisition. *American Journal of Sociology, 80*(4), 871–883.

Van deVliert, E. (1981). A three step theory of role conflict resolution. *Journal of Social Psychology, 113* (1), 77–83.

Chapter 6

Fantasy Patterns of the Pregnant Woman

Fantasy has been viewed as a pleasant diversion, a waste of time, and a key to psychoanalytically defined disturbances; it is even a type of escapist literature. Rarely has it been viewed as an important indicator of a pregnant woman's well-being, providing cues to the woman's concerns and problems requiring intervention from the nurse. Yet fantasy—both daydreams and night dreams—is very prevalent in the mental life of the pregnant woman. Fantasies may reflect great anxiety and fear over the coming birth and imminent mothering of an infant. They may also be vital mechanisms enabling the woman to work through a variety of problem situations.

The focus of this chapter concerns the fantasy state during pregnancy, the role fantasy plays for the pregnant woman, and how fantasy might serve as an indicator for planned nursing intervention at the primary level of health care; namely, that of health maintenance and illness prevention. The schema for classifying fantasies during pregnancy emerged from a fantasy survey (Sherwen, 1981) in which the following question was answered: What is fantasy state like during the third trimester of pregnancy, and, further, what role, if any, could fantasy analysis play in nursing care of the pregnant client? *Fantasy* is here defined as verbal or written reports of all mentation whose ideational products are not evaluated by the individual in terms of usefulness in advancing some immediate goal extrinsic to the mentation itself (Klinger, 1971). In Sherwen's (1981) study, fantasy state includes both daydreams and night dreams, which are considered variants of the same state of mentation (Klinger, 1971; Singer, 1975).

The studies on fantasies during pregnancy cited here will demonstrate what dreams are like during pregnancy. In addition, a suggestion will be offered as to how dreams in pregnancy may be classified according to content and affect, and how nursing interpretations of fantasy might lead to nursing interventions.

FANTASY: AN OVERVIEW

As a concept of interest in health care, fantasy has been largely ignored; however, it did and continues to play a prominent role in the various schools of psychoanalysis from which come most theoretical speculations concerning this entity.

Recently, health care professionals have begun to be interested in fantasy as an indicator of health and to evolve objective measurement tools, contrasting to the Thematic Apperception Test (TAT) and Rorschach Test utilized by the psychoanalyst. Singer and Antrobus (1963), pioneers in this area of tool development, see fantasy in the individual as a result of interactions between a complex processing system involving ever-reverberating content from long-term memory storage and almost continuous processing of input material from the physical and social environment (Singer, 1975). The vividness of the fantasy material, then, becomes dependent on the amount of incoming sensory input. For example, night fantasy materials during sleep (dreams) are frequently vivid due to minimal competing incoming stimuli, while day fantasies (daydreams) are often pale in contrast since sensory channels are being utilized to process visual, auditory, and olfactory material. From this conceptualization, Singer and Antrobus (1963) synthesized a definition of fantasy as a reported train of thought, imagery, or internal monologue that may occur as a shift of attention away from an ongoing task or external perceptual situation. Fantasy may be relatively organized or kaleidoscopic, involve wishful pictures or imagery of frightening possibilites, or be relatively practical, realistic sequences of events or grossly impossible occurrences.

The ability to fantasize has been viewed as a personality trait (Singer, 1975) or a state that may be aroused in an individual. Klinger (1971) has synthesized a picture of the nature of fantasy, and we can apply his ideas to fantasies generated during pregnancy. Through an analysis of materials on dreams and play, both of which seem to be intrinsically related to fantasy, Klinger describes the structure of fantasy. In brief, he believes fantasy is made up of hierarchically ordered shifts in content in the stream of consciousness. The components of fantasy are to be considered as complex amalgamations of responses that constitute states of the entire organism. These response segments can be highly integrated into the human system, yet novel in each circumstance. Changes in fantasy content are due to elicitation of various "subselves" of the human organism. "Current concerns" mediate the subself elicited and the corresponding fantasy state evolved. Other environmental influences can elicit fantasy in Klinger's scheme, and fantasy behavior is loosely related to the individual's pattern of overt behavior.

Another important aspect of fantasy that is alluded to by both Singer (1975) and Klinger (1971) is the fact that, whether one is having day or night fantasies (daydreams or night dreams), one is basically in the same state of consciousness. Singer (1975) has already been cited as saying that the differences between night dreams and daydreams are to be found in the different nature of incoming sensory stimuli. The internal processing traits stay the same during both situations.

Klinger (1971) has evolved a more elaborate set of links between day and night fantasies and in his book supports his conclusions with many studies on night dreams and daydreams, as well as with an analysis of the literature. The links include common structural characteristics for both forms, the fact that both will reflect current concerns, and the fact that both are problem-solving mechanisms. Based on Klinger's and Singer's (1975) conclusions that daydreams and night dreams are parts of a continuous process, both entities will be subsumed under the term *fantasy*.

FANTASY STATE DURING PREGNANCY

This chapter concerns the state of fantasy production during pregnancy. Many studies indicate that fantasy pattern is actually altered during pregnancy. Deutch (1965) believed that feminine anatomy directly affected a woman's fantasy, which, during pregnancy, was said to help her become more and more passive in awaiting motherhood. Benedek (1970) saw fantasy influencing the emotional course of pregnancy and therefore the mother's attitude toward the child. The future mother-child relationship might depend on the woman identifying with and fantasizing about the fetus as the "loving and loved self," a state fortunate for both mother and fetus. Alternatively, she might see it as the "bad, aggressive, devouring self" and fantasize about carrying a monster, resulting in panic or depression. Such fantasies augur poorly for the evolving mother-child relationship.

Similar to Benedek (1970), Caplan (1959) based formulations concerning fantasy during pregnancy on his clinical observations. He also believed that future relations of the mother to her child are a direct continuation of the mother's relation to her fetus and are mirrored in fantasy content. Caplan believed that the first important aspect of infant-to-be representation in fantasy was the age of the fantasized infant. He held that the best maternal-child relationship would result if the mother fantasized the baby as a little baby, and that these daydreams of a young infant were positively emotionally toned. Caplan had found that women who only dream of older children often fear the very young infant as an uncontrollable bundle of instincts.

Another important aspect in pregnant fantasies, to Caplan (1959), was the fantasized sex of the infant. If the mother fantasized infants of both sexes and was indifferent to the sex of her fetus, a positive mother-child relationship was postulated. If the mother consistently fantasized about one sex in the infant, a possible conflict in the maternal-child relationship might be anticipated.

More descriptive information of fantasies in pregnancy came from the clinical observations of Rubin (1972, 1984), who found a discernible fantasy pattern as the pregnancy progressed. Early in pregnancy there were fewer fantasies than there were later on in the pregnancy. In the first trimester, fantasies about the child seemed to stem from outside stimuli, often symbolically linked to pregnancy, such as an egg. During the second and third trimesters, fantasies were more specifically related to what the child would be like when it arrived, and were rich and vivid in content. These fantasies, Rubin believed, served the important function for the woman of physical and psychological "binding-in" to the idea of having her own child. They served to orient her toward the child in the future: its sex, appearance, and personality. Rubin found that, in general, during the second trimester, fantasies about the sex of the child tended to be of infants of either sex. In the third trimester, the sex of the child in fantasy tended to be female. Concerning the age of the fantasized child, Rubin held that the child was always of a size larger than a newborn infant. In mid-pregnancy, the woman tended to fantasize a child in situations of her own recent wished-for adolescent past. This was followed by fantasies of a young, preschool-age child. The smallest-sized child a woman was able to fantasize, according to Rubin, was a child of about six months size. The mother-to-be is said to be unprepared through fantasy for a very small infant at birth.

Rubin (1972, 1984) also collected other descriptive information about the infant. In pregnant women's fantasies, the child was seen as occupying space only through movement and as having a "floating, evanescent, impermanent" quality. Finally, Rubin described fears during pregnancy as they were manifest in fantasy, which she saw as very unpleasant and troublesome. Fantasy in the third trimester was influenced by the imminence of labor, the burdensomeness of the enlarged body, and the sense of decreasing control over the body and its vulnerability. Fantasies at this time were of a hairy, animallike child or of a dismembered or grossly incomplete child. As labor became more imminent, there were increasing fantasies of the woman herself being in dangerous and destructive situations. Rubin saw daydreams and night dreams as being continuous processes, both reflecting changes manifest by the developing stages of pregnancy.

Some other experimental designs have also provided information about fantasy state during pregnancy. Pregnant women's dreams were compared to dreams of nonpregnant female subjects in a study by Van DeCastle and Kindler (1968). When analyzed, the pregnant women's dreams revealed a greater percentage of architectural references. Pregnancy-related concerns, such as doctor appointments, diet, clumsiness, and decreased locomotion, were quite common among the pregnant women, along with the feeling that their husbands found other women more appealing. Dependence-independence conflicts, especially in relation to the pregnant woman's mother, were present in the dreams. Very striking during the last trimester of pregnancy was a great frequency of dreams in the pregnant women dealing with the unborn child, generally occurring in the context of anxiety. The baby was often described as deformed or of unusual size or possessing unusual skills at birth.

Bibring (1959) studied the psychological processes in pregnancy and found unusual projected psychological material in patients in a prenatal clinic. She uncovered "disturbed" thinking, that is, magical thinking, premonitions, depressive reactions, introjection, and paranoid mechanisms. She also did a dream analysis of these individuals and found a high incidence of apprehension, along with images of misfortune occurring to the dreamer and the unborn child.

Winget and Kapp (1972) theorized that fears and anxiety about delivery and the role of motherhood would be a contributing cause in prolonged labor when there were no medical reasons for this condition. In their study, they attempted to circumvent ego defenses and get at fear and anxiety through the medium of night dreams. The investigators elicited night dream recollections through interviews with 100 "healthy" primigravidas and then assessed the lengths of their labor. The women were divided into three groups: Group I, having labor of less than 10 hours; Group II, having labor of 10 to 20 hours; and Group III, having over 20 hours in labor. Results were significant in several areas. There was a relation ($p < .01$) between frequency of dreams with anxiety in manifest content and the duration of childbirth. Members of Group I had the highest percent (80%) of anxiety in dream reports, while members of Group III had the lowest percent (25%). The same pattern was found with themes of threat, although somewhat attenuated. Also, the more mobility or movement found in night dreams, the shorter the labor. The authors concluded that, near the end of pregnancy, pregnant women normally have fears. The presence of anxiety and threatening themes in night dreams was seen as an attempt to master in fantasy anticipatory stress in waking life, thus pointing to the problem-solving capabilities of fantasy.

Gillman (1968) also investigated night dreams to see how the experience of pregnancy was reflected. His research consisted of analyzing night dream reports from 44 pregnant women and comparing them to dreams of a control group of nonpregnant college women. In comparison to 1 percent of the nonpregnant group, 40 percent of the pregnant group had dreams about a baby. Fifty percent of pregnant women, compared to 10 percent of nonpregnant women, had dreams with themes of misfortune, harm, and environmental threats. In addition, 12 percent of the pregnant group reported dreams of crippled and deformed infants, and 75 percent of this group had dreams with an emotional tone of apprehension.

Finally, Sherwen (1980), in a study designed to validate Singer's Imaginal Processes Inventory (1966) on a sample of pregnant women, demonstrated a different fantasy profile on the inventory subscales for pregnant than for nonpregnant women. Pregnant women had a much higher frequency (p = .0001) of night dreaming than did nonpregnant women. In addition, nonpregnant women had a much higher frequency (p = .009) of problem-solving fantasies than did pregnant women in a Lamaze class group.

From the preceding studies on fantasy during the pregnant state, two generalizations may be made. First, fantasy is different in pregnant than in non-pregnant states and, second, fantasy during pregnancy, especially during the third trimester, can be highly negative and troublesome in nature.

FANTASY AND ACCEPTANCE OF THE MATERNAL ROLE

In the preceding chapter, it was seen that fantasy, according to both Rubin (1984) and Lederman (1984), is vital in the process necessary for assuming the maternal role and also for acceptance of the pregnancy in general. Rubin (1984) sees fantasy as one of the necessary phases a woman passes through in the process of attaining a maternal identity. Fantasy marks the beginning of "internalization" of the maternal role, whereby the mother-to-be, through imagery, projects how it will be to mother a child in the future. To Rubin, "fantasies are instrumental in the binding-in . . . to self as mother" (p. 30). Rubin also sees fantasy as a necessary component in resolving grief for loss of the past life and for the roles a woman must give up. Fantasy allows a woman to review her past in memory and recognize that these past stages are irreversibly finished.

Lederman (1984) sees fantasy as a major form of preparation for motherhood. This preparation occurs in three initial steps:

1. Envisioning oneself as mother
2. Thinking about those characteristics one wishes to have as a mother
3. Anticipating future life changes that will be necessary

Lederman sees dreaming as a process not sharply differentiated from fantasy. In Lederman's subjects, reported dream content tended to parallel actual concerns. Five categories of dreams commonly occurred: schools dreams, reliving childhood, motherhood/career conflicts, confidence in maternal skills, and food/infant intactness dreams.

These themes pointed to areas that must be resolved by the pregnant woman in order for her to accept her pregnancy and move into the maternal role.

FANTASY AND PROBLEM SOLVING DURING PREGNANCY

Many theoreticians and investigators have pointed to the role of fantasy in helping the pregnant woman to solve potential crises in her current and future life.

Levy and McGee (1975) looked at crisis resolution through fantasy production as an attribute that might affect the individual during labor. These investigators, defining labor and delivery as a crisis, attempted to study the woman's ability to resolve crisis in fantasy, plus attitudes concerning childbirth inherited from her own mother, as determinants of a positive childbirth experience. Levy and McGee based their work on the theory that fear arousal in certain amounts has a "psychological inoculation" effect that will enable the individual to understand and deal with the stressful event better by imagining the event and resolving it in fantasy. Thus, those pregnant women, especially primigravidas, exposed to moderate descriptions of labor and delivery from their mothers, will deal better with their own labor and delivery than women receiving no information concerning labor and delivery, or women receiving either very positive or negative descriptions of labor and delivery. With a normal, moderate exposure to realistic labor and delivery fears, the woman can do the "work of worry" through fantasy production and have an imaginative rehearsal concerning labor and delivery. She will be able, through fantasy, to envision the possible outcomes of her labor and delivery. In her imaginings, she will be able to solve a variety of problems and devise solutions to alternative outcomes of the labor and delivery process. For example, she will be able to imagine a labor where she has fetal monitoring, including how she will act; or she may imagine a labor that is truly controlled by Lamaze techniques.

If communications concerning this process are absent or of a very positive nature, the woman will tend to deny the stressful situation and will be at a disadvantage when faced with the crisis of labor and delivery. She will be unable to imagine anything but a "perfect" labor and delivery. If communications are too negative, the woman will be immobilized and too fearful for a realistic imaginative appraisal of her labor. Levy & McGee (1975) found that these conjectures held under experimental conditions with a sample of 60 primigravidas. Thus, it seems necessary for fantasy, with its components of imaginative rehearsal and problem solving, to be encouraged during pregnancy.

A SCHEMA FOR CLASSIFYING FANTASIES DURING PREGNANCY

Although surveys and research have added greatly to the theory of fantasy during pregnancy, fantasy has not been seen as a basis for nursing intervention in a systematic manner. One important outcome of the study of fantasy in pregnancy would be development of a categorization or schema that would aid the nurse in counseling her pregnant client.

In 1980, Sherwen did a survey of fantasies experienced by pregnant women in their third trimester (Sherwen, 1981). This fantasy study of third-trimester primigravidas was done as part of a larger experimental study of fantasy state in pregnancy during the third trimester (Sherwen, 1980). In addition to responding to the experimental questionnaires, volunteers were asked to record any night dreams or daydreams they had had during the testing interval (approximately five weeks). As mentioned earlier, day and night dreams are considered as variants of the same state of mentation and so both forms of fantasy production were considered necessary.

Although a total of 153 pregnant women were included in the larger experimental study, the third-trimester fantasy study was begun after approximately one-third of the large study's sample of women had been tested with the experimental questionnaires. This survey of fantasies was in response to spontaneous requests made by the subjects to record their night dreams and daydreams and discuss them with the investigator during the home visits made to collect data. Subjects seemed to perceive discussion of and support about their fantasies as important to their total well-being.

Of the approximately 100 third-trimester primigravidas surveyed, 50 recorded at least one day or night dream. The total of recorded fantasies was 89. The 50 individuals were between the ages of 20 and 30, of mixed race and ethnic background, and of middle-class socioeconomic status. When the fantasies of these individuals were examined, they seemd to fall naturally into categories or groupings. It was poss-ible to develop a classification schema of third-trimester fantasies based on the following principles:

1. The *content* of the day and night dream. This might give clues as to the current concerns of the pregnant woman.
2. Verbal and nonverbal *communications* of the pregnant woman dur-ing the discussion of the day or night dream. This might give in-sight into the affective state or feeling tone the woman has con-cerning the dream. A woman might communicate positive or negative feelings about a particular fantasy.
3. *Verification* by the pregnant woman concerning the current con-cerns that might be the basis of a fantasy, and how she feels about them.

The classification schema, that was developed from these principles is shown in Table 6–1. Such a classification schema is, of course, incom-plete and needs further verification from additional studies of fantasy state in pregnancy. In addition, it deals only with third-trimester fan-tasies, which, while they are the most vivid and disturbing of all fan-tasies produced during pregnancy, are certainly not representative of fantasy state during pregnancy as a whole.

THIRD-TRIMESTER FANTASY WORK AND NURSING INTERVENTIONS

Although somewhat premature at this point, this classification schema might give a framework for conceptualizing third-trimester fantasies and for aiding nursing interventions, upon assessment and diagnosis of the concerns expressed by the pregnant client. Nursing intervention in response to fantasy assessment can be seen as a form of primary-level health care intervention. In this light, both positive trends (such as problem-solving fantasies) and problem trends (such as decrease in bonding fantasies) can be identified and either supported or altered. The following are some examples of the ways in which I have inter-vened in these areas.

Table 6-1. Classification of Third-Trimester Fantasies

Content	Affect (feeling tone)
1. Everyday fantasies (38% of fantasies). Examples:	
a. Characteristics of infant-to-be (sex, looks, hair, eyes); baby at different stages of growth and development; living with and caring for baby (playing, feeding, loving)	Positive
b. Reaction of husband, significant others, to infant	Pos. and/or neg.
2. Being attacked (mother or symbol) (21% of fantasies). Examples: Burglar stealing; intruders in house; falling down stairs	Negative
3. Giving birth to an "abnormal" infant (12% of fantasies). Examples:	
a. Misshappen or deformed; abnormal size, age, or ability	Negative
b. Multiple infants (usually twins)	Positive
4. Restoration (11% of fantasies). Examples: Death (resolve past deaths, complete intergenerational cycle); reparation (make amends with family, friends)	Positive
5. Sexuality (8% of fantasies). Examples:	
a. Sexual relations with husband, mate	Positive
b. Sexual relations with others (father-in-law, obstetrician)	Negative
6. Being inside; drowning (5% of fantasies). Examples: Subway tunnels; sinking in lake of slush	Negative
7. Losing or forgetting (2.5% of fantasies). Examples: Baby, others	Negative
8. Being unprepared (2.5% of fantasies). Examples: Exams, labor	Negative
9. Symbols frequently found. Examples:	
a. Water (lakes, ocean, rivers, rain, swimming pools, drinks)	Pos. and/or neg.
b. Stairs, especially spiral	Negative
c. Animals (baby animals, pets; often in threatening situations)	Negative
d. Bright or drab colors	Neg. and/or pos.

Supporting and Enhancing Positive Fantasies

The nurse can support and enhance trends toward positive fantasy responses to pregnancy, labor, and delivery. The following night dream provides an example of a fantasy whose content might be supported by the nurse:

> "I have had one bad nightmare in the last week. I dreamt that my husband and I were in his car about to go through a car wash. For some reason, my husband got out of the car and I went through the car wash in his car alone. At the end of the car wash, the car with me inside dropped off into a deep lake of snowy slush. I spent the rest of the dream trying to figure out how to get out of the car without drowining, freezing to death, or suffocating. I awoke before I was killed or saved. I remained levelheaded and unpanicked while I tried to figure a way out of my dilemma."

Although basically quite a negative fantasy, this night dream demonstrates one very positive trend in the primigravida's repertoire for dealing with her pregnancy and impending labor. Even though she is literally all alone in her dream, abandoned by her husband and "drowning" in a lake of slush, she sees herself dealing with the situation in a calm, problem-solving manner. The feeling associated with the dream is not totally negative, as the tone is hopeful, one of "solving problems." In a counseling situation, it would be vital to support this woman's use of a problem-solving attitude in dealing with the aspects of labor and delivery that frighten her. In this case, specific suggestions of how to solve the possible problem of getting her husband in a more supportive role were explored, such as mutual involvement in parenting classes and preparation activities for the infant-to-be. It was suggested she enroll in a Lamaze or other childbirth preparation class, and she was given reading lists concerning the process of labor and delivery. These interventions supported this primigravida's strivings to solve problems in an independent manner.

Ameliorating Excessive Negativity or Fear

The nurse can reduce the impact of excessively negative or unrealistically frightened fantasies by "defusing" a frightening fantasy situation and by supplying realistic information about a situation or impending event.

"Frightened" fantasies in the pregnant woman can be handled on several levels. First, it is important to remember that all negative-toned fantasies are not "bad." Fantasies that deal realistically with potential problems in pregnancy, labor, and delivery, and with the infant-to-be, are actually beneficial for the pregnant woman. It has been found that women who imaginatively rehearse how they would handle potential problems in the upcoming events, for example having a Cesarean delivery actually handle all events better than women who have had only positive fantasies about the infant and the labor and delivery experience. Fantasy production that is too positive or too negative can leave the parturient unprepared for the real event of labor and delivery, and for caring for a newborn (Levy & McGee, 1975).

Fantasies in the "being attacked" category in the schema can provide examples of how to intervene to prevent potential problems resulting from too negative a fantasy state. The first technique is to ascertain the actual area of concern, since many fantasies utilize symbols instead of direct representation of the event. When the concern is identified, it can be "defused" by discussing it with the pregnant woman in realistic terms. At this point, the second technique is used—supplying realistic information about the situation or event and allowing the woman to resolve her fear in her own manner.

For example, one primigravida had this night dream:

> "A vampire was attacking many people at random. I was not in any immediate danger. All I could do was watch . . . "

This fantasy had a highly negative tone and used symbols. The theme was definitely one of being "attacked" and "drained" by something evil. Distancing mechanisms were used, since others, not the primigravida herself, were being attacked and she was not in "immediate danger." However, a sense of being helpless in the situation was also implied, since she could only watch. Thus, the associated feeling was negative. Upon discussion, it became evident that this primigravida's concern was the potentially intrusive procedures that might be done during labor and delivery (that is, the enema, episiotomy, and internal examinations) and her feelings of being unable to protect herself from them. Identification and discussion of the fearful situations helped to defuse her fears.

The primigravida was then ready for the second phase: being supplied with realistic information about the events she feared. The procedures that might be done and the rationale for doing each were discussed in depth. Pros and cons of each intrusive procedure were weighed by the woman, with the nurse as an information source and sounding board. This primigravida, after understanding the procedures, resolved her fears by deciding to discuss with her obstetrician her wishes not to have an enema or an episiotomy unless absolutely necessary.

Observing the Progress of "Bonding" Clues in Fantasy

Rubin (1984) and others have pointed to fantasies about the infant-to-be and caring for the baby as important to the process of "binding-in" the infant to the mother and family. The fantasy production in the "everyday fantasy" category provides a measure of the progress of the bonding process before the actual birth of the infant. Here, the most important observation to make in problem prevention would be the suppression of these fantasies. Inability to fantasize at all about the infant—including the possible sex and other characteristics, as well as nurturing the baby—is one important clue to a potential "bonding risk."

For example, several nursing students whom I clinically supervised reported fantasies of this nature among their patients. One patient, in her eighth month of pregnancy, repeatedly referred to her infant-to-be as "it." The woman further refused to imagine how she would care for the infant and verbalized an inability to picture her child and a lack of interest in whether her child would be a boy or girl. Her nonverbal communications were overtly hostile when queried on her impending motherhood, and she said that she "couldn't imagine herself being the mother of a crying kid." At this point, it would be vital to look for potential blocks to bonding, such as unresolved grief or loss, marital instability, role ambivalence, and so forth. In this woman's case, an examination of her family history revealed that she had been abandoned early in the pregnancy by the father of the infant-to-be.

If a tangible block can be discovered, the nurse can intervene to resolve this crisis situation or, if the problem is too complex to deal with, the nurse can refer to a clinical specialist in nursing or another professional. However, identification of the potential problem through fantasy production and support through more intense intervention is the responsibility of every nurse involved with prenatal care. I did not discover anyone in the current sample who was repressing "everyday fantasies" and so did not actually intervene in this area.

Encouraging Preparation for Childbirth

The nurse can provide, through fantasy, educational and other help for the client in her preparatory activities. This form of nursing intervention is similar to that used to work with someone with a frightening fantasy, but it does not require the "defusing" phase. Among my clients, there were several fantasies that were not frightening per se but spoke specifically to the parturient's not being ready for the upcoming events. These fantasies had associated feelings that were definitely negatively toned and thus required intervention. These were grouped into a category called "being unprepared." The following is an example:

> "[I have had] recurring dreams of being unprepared for final exams at college or high school. Feelings of panic because no work has been done all semester."

Again, symbolism was used, but the overall thrust was unmistakably "not being prepared," while the associated feeling tone was negative. Nursing intervention was simple for this primigravida. After discussing her concern about being ready for labor and delivery, her plans to take Lamaze childbirth-preparation classes were examined. She concluded, with support, that childbirth-preparation classes were an important mechanism to prepare her for the event, especially since they would give her actual "work" to do in preparation (that is, reading and practicing the exercises). In addition, I suggested several books and pamphlets that would help her begin her preparation process and give her work in the present.

Alleviating Guilt Feelings

Guilt feelings generally fall into two categories: sexual encounters and ambivalent feelings concerning the infant. Fantasies falling into the sexuality category are further divided into two basic kinds: those fantasies dealing with a sexual encounter with a person who is perceived by the pregnant woman as legitimate (such as a husband), and those fantasies dealing with persons perceived as not legitimate (such as a father-in-law). While both types of fantasy deal with sex, the first variety of sexual fantasy seems to have a highly positive affective tone and is a source of pleasure to the pregnant woman. The second type, however, is problematic, since the pregnant woman usually feels guilty for fantasizing a sexual relation with someone perceived as socially unacceptable. In this case, the associated feeling tone is negative. Counseling in this instance deals with the alleviation of guilt, since sexual fantasies, especially night dreams, are quite common to pregnant women. Helping the woman to realize that her dreams are not abnormal and that she is not alone in having such fantasies while pregnant is often sufficient to alleviate associated guilt.

Fantasies from another category in the schema, "losing/forgetting," also seemed to induce guilt feelings in the pregnant woman. These fantasies, usually night dreams, had themes about losing or forgetting the infant-to-be. The following is an example of one primigravida's night dream:

> " . . . doing routine activities and forgetting about the baby: I go out and then remember the baby."

This woman, when the dream was discussed, expressed some minor ambivalence, not so much about the baby itself, but of her impending role of "mother." I told her that this was a common concern of mothers-to-be, and we discussed coping strategies for parents of newborns and the possibility of her joining a new parents' group. This proved to be a successful intervention.

Supporting "Restoration" Efforts

Interventions based on fantasies in the final category to be discussed, "restoration," are supportive in nature, since the trend revealed in these day and night dreams seems to be highly positive. Of the 50 individuals recording day and night dreams, 11% had fantasies falling in this category. As Caplan (1959) believed, it would seem that the woman has a chance during pregnancy to rework old crises and, as it were, make her intergenerational pattern complete. These women had fantasies about dead and lost friends and relatives and seemed to resolve or repair the loss through the impending birth of the infant. The process was almost like a generational "linking-up" of the infant-to-be with ancestors. One example of a nightdream in this category follows:

> "I had one in which . . . I was pushing my newborn baby in a baby carriage. I passed large groups of people sitting on long, long benches. One of these people was an uncle of mine who had died two years ago. He winked and smiled at me. The overall feeling was happy but rather anxious and tense, sort of like being late for an important professional appointment."

Here, the intergenerational linking-up is evident, with the dead uncle approving of the baby-to-be. The positive feeling tone of the dream is apparent.

Another night dream described by a different woman falls in this category and illustrates the trend toward resolution of death of a loved one. This primigravida had lost a younger brother, age 14, five years previous to her pregnancy:

> " . . . [I] dreamt about my brother learning to have fun in camp. I knew he was going to die, but he was having fun in the pool with his instructor and it didn't bother me. [Later I] dreamt about my brother seeing a Russian psychiatrist, letting his feelings out in sweet breath. [It] didn't bother me that I knew he was dying, because he was being let loose by talking to [the] psychiatrist."

Both this woman and the woman described earlier in this section had fantasies with an obviously positive affective state and were therefore supported in the process of further exploration of these feelings. This type of fantasy may well be an important mechanism for resolving unfinished grieving processes connected with death and loss, and for binding the infant into the total extended and lineal family system.

SUMMARY

The foregoing examples have illustrated how conceptual groupings or categories of fantasy state in pregnancy, plus the feeling tone of day and night dream reports, may serve as one basis for determining nursing intervention for the pregnant woman. As with any other type of assessment, it is only justified when taken in concert with other areas of assessment and put into the context of the whole. Because fantasy in pregnancy is something obvious and often disturbing to the pregnant woman, it cannot be ignored by nurses who wish to care for the whole individual. More important, it may serve as an indicator that will enable the nurse to get at vital core concerns of the parturient and to intervne at a health-maintenance/illness-prevention level.

REFERENCES

Benedek, T. (1970). The psychology of pregnancy. In A. Benedek & T. Benedek (Eds.), *Parenthood*. Boston: Little, Brown.

Bibring, G. L. (1959). Some consideration of the psychological processes in pregnancy. *The Psychoanalytic Study of the Child, 15,* 113–121.

Caplan, G. (1959). *Concepts of mental health and consultation.* Washington DC: U.S. Department of Health Education and Welfare.

Deutch, H. (1965). *The psychology of women.* New York: Grune and Stratton.

Gillman, R. (1968). The dreams of pregnant women and maternal adaptation. *The American Journal of Orthopsychiatry, 38*(4), 688–692.

Klinger, E. (1971). *The structure and function of fantasy.* New York: Wiley Interscience.

Lederman, R. (1984). *Psychosocial adaptation in pregnancy.* Englewood Cliffs, NJ: Prentice-Hall.

Levy, J., & McGee, R. (1975). Childbirth as a crisis: A test of Janis theory of communication and stress resolution. *Journal of Personality and Social Psychology, 31*(1), 171–179.

Rubin, R. (1972). Fantasy and object constancy in maternal relationships. *MCN, The Maternal-Child Nursing Journal, 1*(2), 101–111.

Rubin, R. (1984). *Maternal identity and the maternal experience.* New York: Springer.

Sherwen, L. (1980). *An investigation into the effects of psychoprophylactic method training and locus of control on fantasy production and body cathexis in the primiparous woman.* Unpublished doctoral dissertation, New York University.

Sherwen, L. (1981). Fantasies during the third trimester of pregnancy. *MCN-The American Journal of Maternal Child Nursing, 6*(6), 398–401.

Singer, A., & Antrobus, J. (1963). A factor analytic study of daydreaming and conceptually-related cognitive and personality variables. *Perceptual and Motor Skills, Monograph Supplement, 17*(3).

Singer, J. (1966). *Imaginal processes inventory.* Princeton, N.J.: Educational Testing Services.

Singer, J. (1975). Navigating the stream of consciousness. *American Psychologist, 65,* 720.

Van DeCastle, R., & Kindler, P. (1968). Dream content during pregnancy. *Psychophysiology, 4,*375.

Winget, C., & Kapp, F. (1972). The relation of manifest content of dreams to duration of childbirth in primiparae. *Psychosomatic Medicine, 34*(4), 313–320.

Chapter 7

Body Image in Pregnancy

Ellen Schuzman

Pregnancy is characterized by rapidly occurring body changes with psychological and sociological implications (Bibring, Dwyer, Huntington, & Valenstein, 1961). Often pregnancy is described as a developmental process in which the pregnant woman is confronted with psychological tasks that correspond to the somatic and physiological changes (Budd, 1977; Tanner, 1969). Adjustment of one's body image in pregnancy is an ongoing task dealt with by the pregnant woman. This chapter focuses on the relationship of body image to the psychological well-being of the pregnant woman. Changes in the pregnant woman's body image, as reflective of the psychological and somatic changes, will be examined. The chapter will also present some of the behavioral manifestations of the pregnant woman's evolving body image. Nursing strategies for helping the pregnant woman evolve a healthy body image will be identified.

THE CONCEPT OF BODY IMAGE

Humans are open systems, continuously interacting with their environment. As a manifestation of this interaction between an individual and the environment, the individual's body image, a perceptual awareness and attitude concerning the pattern and organization of one's body, evolves (Norris, 1978; Schilder, 1970). Body image encompasses the complex process of gathering, evaluating, and reacting to information about one's body, its parts, and its environment (Norris, 1978; Schilder, 1970). The body image consists of stored psychological, physiological, and sociological experiences that serve as reference points, collectively called body schema, for incoming perceptions and attitude formation (Schilder, 1970). Changes in the body, a body part, or the environment should result in an augmented body image.

As the individual grows and develops, the body image is formed. The process is gradual until the period of preadolescence and adolescence, when there are multiple psychosocial and physiological changes (Dempsey, 1972; Murray, 1972; Petrella, 1978; Weinberg, 1978). The mature body image is the successful outcome of the integrative process in which rapid body changes are incorporated into the body schema (Schilder, 1970). However, when an individual with a mature body image experiences a threat to self or is trying to deal with illness, disease, or loss of a body part, anxiety, fear, and body image disturbances may result (Corbreil, 1971; Kolb, 1959; Leonard, 1972; Murray, 1972).

During pregnancy the body undergoes rapid change, and the psychological and sociological implications of this require adjustment of the body image (Budd, 1977; Fawcett, 1977, 1978; Moore, 1978; Rubin, 1968; Tanner, 1969; Weinberg, 1978). Generally, the changes in the pregnant woman's body image follow a developmental pattern and may be observed in specific behaviors. A review of the literature reveals that both the perceptual and attitudinal/affective domains of body image are altered in pregnancy.

THE PERCEPTUAL DOMAIN

Studies concerning the perceptual domain that have relevance to pregnancy focus upon the following body image subconcepts: body awareness, body-image distortion, body boundaries, body size, and body space. The following literature discussed includes both qualitative and quantitative approaches to studying these body image subconcepts.

Body Awareness

The most overt and marked physical changes during pregnancy are in the size and shape of the uterus and abdomen. Positive signs of pregnancy include the presence of quickening, an audible fetal heart beat, and palpable fetal parts. Yet long before the woman looks pregnant, long before there are positive outward signs of pregnancy, the woman knows or suspects she is pregnant. The woman's body image picks up on physical cues of amenorrhea, nausea, fatigue, and breast tenderness. No matter how slight the stimulus, the woman attempts to use the clue to validate the pregnancy (Rubin, 1970).

The pregnant woman in her first trimester begins to focus in on her self and her body; she begins to heighten her awareness of bodily changes. Bibring et al.'s (1961) intensive analytic study of 15 primigravidas throughout their pregnancies indicated that during the first trimester the woman is narcissistic. Colman and Colman (1971), through clinical practice, found that beginning in the first trimester and peaking in the third trimester the pregnant woman becomes introverted and passive. The narcissism, introversion, and passivity allow the woman time and energy to focus in on the multiple body changes and incorporate the change into her body image. Bibring et al. (1961) noted that, during the first trimester, awareness of the somatic changes causes the woman to view the fetus as a foreign object that is invading her body. This creates psychological upheaval. To cope with this turmoil, the pregnant woman incorporates the fetus into her body image and views the fetus as an extension of self. Tanner's (1969) descriptive research on psychological tasks of pregnancy supports the findings of Bibring et al. (1961). Specifically, Tanner (1969) found that, in the first trimester, primigravida women had increased interest and concern about bodily and mood changes and expressed more positive interest and awareness of changes than later in pregnancy. Additionally, Tannner found that in the first trimester women viewed the fetus as a "thing" in terms of the actual stage of fetal development. Tanner concluded, as Bibring et al. (1961) did, that during the first trimester, as they focus on the body changes, women tend to view the fetus as an extension of self and not as a separate entity.

As the woman becomes aware of more overt signs of pregnancy, her body image changes. Bibring et al. (1961) noted that the second trimester event of quickening disrupts the narcissistic process and stimulates the woman to view the fetus as separate from her body. The pregnant woman begins to prepare for her role as mother and for anatomical separation from the fetus. Tanner (1969), similarly noting that by the second trimester women described their fetus as an infant, outside of self, concluded that beginning in the second trimester the woman readjusts her body image to view the fetus as a separate being. Tanner (1969), Rubin (1970), and Caplan (1961) also attribute the overt changes in body configuration, size, and shape, along with the feelings associated with these changes, to the alterations that the body image undergoes. Specifically, Tanner (1969) and Rubin (1970) note that the enlarging body, particularly the abdomen/uterus, tells the woman and others that she is pregnant. In the second trimester the woman begins to wear maternity clothes out of necessity rather than for validation (Rubin, 1970).

By the third trimester, however, the woman's enlarged abdomen/ uterus contributes to a feeling of disenchantment and a perception of her pregnant body as almost discontinous with her nonpregnant state. The woman, at this point, wants the pregnancy to end. She actively prepares for the physical, anatomical separation from the fetus. Preparing baby items and baby clothes, attending childbirth classes, making plans for the trip to the hospital, and deciding on which method to use for feeding the baby are behavioral indications that the pregnant woman now views the fetus as a separate entity.

The literature discussed thus far indicates that during pregnancy there is an increased awareness in one's body and body parts. Some studies have been undertaken to explore body awareness during pregnancy directly, while other studies indirectly shed light on this issue. The Body Prominence Test (Fisher, 1970) has been used to assess the amount of body awareness in the general population. This instrument asks each subject to write down 20 things that he or she is aware of presently. The number of direct or indirect body references are calculated according to a specified protocol. Comparing scores on the Body Prominence Test for pregnant and nonpregnant women, Fisher (1973b) found that the degree of body awareness is not increased for pregnant women. Ruggieri, Milizia, and Romano (1979) also note that, in a sample of 20 third-trimester women and 20 nonpregnant women, pregnancy did not influence the scores on the Body Prominence Test. In contrast, Karmel (1975) found differences in the general amount of body awareness for 32 pregnant women, during the third trimester and 6 weeks postpartum, as compared with 28 nonpregnant control subjects tested over a similar time frame. Using the Body Prominence Test, Karmel (1975) found that the level of body awareness is higher during pregnancy than when not pregnant and that after parturition there is a significant decrease in the the Body Prominence score (p < 0.01).

In the same study, Karmel (1975) also used the Stomach Focus dimension of the Body Focus Questionnaire (Fisher, 1970) to assess body awareness. The Body Focus Questionnaire presents each subject with a series of verbal references to paired body areas; each subject is asked to indicate which of the two body parts stands out most clearly in her or his awareness. Karmel (1975) found significantly higher Stomach Focus scores for pregnant women, when compared to nonpregnant women (p < 0.01). In addition, Karmel found a decrease in Body Focus scores after parturition (p < 0.01). Testing 55 black women and 30 white women during the first and third trimesters and at six weeks postpartum, Harris (1979) found that subjects' scores on the Stomach Focus dimension of the Body Focus Questionnaire changed during pregnancy; specifically, awareness of the stomach peaked at nine months and then was reduced after parturition. However, Harris also found that there were certain predictors for the amount of focus on the stomach: (1) the greater the fetal activity, the greater the focus on the abdomen; (2) for white women, the less active they perceive themselves to be at three months, the greater the stomach awareness at nine months; and (3) for black women, the more afraid they were at three months, the greater the stomach awareness at nine months.

The studies by Karmel (1975) and Harris (1979) directly lend support to the findings of Bibring et al. (1961) and Tannner (1969) which indicate that body awareness is increased during pregnancy and diminishes after parturition. The findings by Fisher (1973b) and Ruggieri et al. (1979) fail to support the statement that body awareness is increased during pregnancy. The latter two studies did not follow subjects over any period of time, while Bibring et al. (1961), Tanner (1969), Karmel (1975), and Harris (1979) followed subjects and controls through part of the pregnancy and the postpartum period. This major difference in methodology may have contributed to the differences in the findings. In addition, the research by Karmel (1975) and Harris (1979) lends supports to Tanner's (1969) and Colman and Colman's (1971) findings suggesting that particular areas of the body (e.g., the stomach) may be focused upon during pregnancy.

Tolar and Digrazia (1977) indirectly lend support to the viewpoint that during pregnancy body awareness or awareness of certain body parts is heightened. Human figure drawings done by 216 women, divided into four groups based on trimester of pregnancy and six-week postpartum status, were compared with respect to each other and with respect to drawings done by 76 nonpregnant gynecological patients. The drawings were analyzed in terms of nine characteristics: clothing, sexual organs, omissions, distortion of the body, open versus closed body parts, size, shading, differentiation, and overall quality. The analysis revealed that, for the most part, the drawings were not distinguishable by trimesters or by postpartum status. A comparison between the 216 pregnant women and 76 nonpregnant women, however, revealed that pregnant women more frequently drew a nude figure ($p < .02$), emphasized sexual organs ($p < .001$), drew distorted figures ($p < .05$), and tended to make figures small in size ($.05 < p > .10$). Tolar and Digrazia interpreted these findings from a psychoanalytic viewpoint that stressed pathology; thus, they made the following negative statements:

1. The high frequency of nude drawings suggest body narcissism, sexual maladjustment, schizoid or introverted tendencies, and preoccupations with bodily processes.
2. Distortion and smallness of the figures indicate low-self esteem and a low energy level.
3. Emphasis on sexual organs suggests sexual preoccupation.

Whether or not one agrees with the grim interpretation of the data presented by Tolar and Digrazia, the findings do suggest that during pregnancy specific components of the body may become focused upon and even distorted.

Fisher (1973a) noted that a body part that fails to meet an individual's expectation of size may become a focus of anxiety. When individuals are concerned or anxious about the body, a high amount of body awareness should be manifested (Secord, 1953). Accordingly, Schuzman (1980) hypothesized that pregnant women who were diagnosed as having a uterus that was smaller than expected in size (i.e., when the distance from the symphysis pubis to the uterine fundus was smaller than expected for a given period of gestation by two centimeters or more) would manifest a higher degree of body awareness than pregnant women with a uterus normal in size for their dates. Using the Body Prominence Test, Schuzman (1980) found that 68% of 19 subjects with a medically diagnosed uterus small in size for dates had a high degree of body awareness, compared to 42% of the 19 subjects with a uterus normal in size. Additionally, the women from both groups who evaluated their uterus as small in size demonstrated a higher degree of body awareness. These findings indicate that the general level of body awareness in pregnancy may be heightened when the uterine size is not appropriate for dates or when the pregnant woman's perception of uterine size is distorted.

Distortion of the Body Image

During pregnancy, the woman's usual sense of well-being frequently is altered. In the first trimester, it may be replaced with nausea, vomiting, fatigue, emotional lability, uncertainty, and a need to withdraw from nonsignificant persons. In the second and third trimesters, the woman is overtly confronted with the pronounced changes in body weight, body configuration, and internal body sensations. By the third trimester the woman may feel awkward when walking and performing activities of daily living. She may experience backaches, stress incontinence, and other bodily discomfort. Furthermore, along with labor and delivery come a wide variety of new body experiences including forceful contractions and perineal pressure, vaginal discharge of fluids, numbness, and decreased control over bodily functions due to anesthesia and the labor and delivery process. The woman may perceive her pregnant body and body parts as alien and incongruent with her usual body image. Leonard (1972) notes that an individual may sense a threat to self when there are severe and rapid body changes, and this certainly may apply to the pregnant woman. Body-image distortion may result whenever there is a threat to self. However, as the research yet to be discussed indicates, a small amount of body-image distortion normally occurs during pregnancy and is generally not problematic.

A study by Uddenberg and Hakansan (1972) demonstrated that psychological variables influence whether or not, and in what manner, distortions in body image will occur. Using aniseikonic glasses, which visually produce a body distortion, Uddenberg and Hakansan found that the more conflicts a person had regarding reproductive functioning the less she or he would perceive any distortion in the pelvic region. The researchers explain that, when there is anxiety associated with a body part, an individual wearing aniseikonic glasses is less likely to perceive distortion of that body part. The lack of distortion experienced may reflect the use of avoidance as a defense mechanism. In contrast, these researchers note that, when a body part receives increased attention as a result of a somatizing tendency, there is likely to be an increased distortion of that body part. In particular, Uddenberg and Hakansan found that women with marked nausea tended to distort their abdomens, while women without nausea reported little distortion. The findings indicate that a small amount of body-image distortion normally occurs during pregnancy, but marked distortion may indicate increased focus upon a body part beyond what is normally encountered during pregnancy. Furthermore, the absence of body-image distortion perception when one has tried to induce a distortion may indicate that the individual is highly anxious about the body or a body part.

Fisher (1973b), Karmel (1975), and Harris (1979) studied body-image distortion in pregnancy, using the Body Distortion Questionnaire (Fisher, 1970). The questionnaire consists of 82 statements that represent seven categories of possible distortion: (1) larger, (2) smaller, (3) boundary, (4) blocked openings, (5) skin, (6) dirt, and (7) depersonalization. Each subject responds to the statement with "yes," "no," or "undecided." The score is obtained by adding the total "yes" and "undecided" responses. The higher the score, the greater the body-image distortion.

Fisher (1973b) found that the number and specific categories of distorted body experiences were high for pregnant women but not significantly different from nonpregnant women. However when the scores for the pregnant women were compared to the same subjects' scores one month postpartum, Fisher found that the total number of distortions in body feelings significantly declined from the pregnant to the nonpregnant state. Fisher suggests the data indicate that (1) for the average woman the marked changes of pregnancy do not produce a significant body-image disturbance and (2) the woman feels more comfortable about her body one month postpartum.

Both Karmel (1975) and Harris (1979) similarly found that the body-image distortion scores fell in the postpartum period; however, Karmel (1975) found that, late in pregnancy, the pregnant women had a significantly higher total score than the nonpregnant control group. Harris (1979) also reported that body-image distortion increased throughout pregnancy, peaking at nine months in black subjects. In contrast, Karmel (1975) found that, for white subjects, body-image distortion decreased throughout the pregnancy. Different predictors of

the degree of body distortion at nine months for black and white subjects were identified by Harris (1979). First, for white subjects, the less
active the pregnancy was perceived to be, the more distortion there was.
Second, the less ready the white subjects were to assume the role of
motherhood, the greater the body-image distortion. Finally, for black
women, the more positive their attitude toward self, the less body-
image distortion.

Drawing conclusions from the research by Uddenberg & Hakansan
(1972), Fisher (1973b), Karmel (1975), and Harris (1979), one should
expect some body-image distortion during pregnancy; however,
marked distortion may be indicative of a severe body-image disturbance, marked bodily concern, growing conflicts over reproductive
functioning, difficulties in assuming the mothering role, and a negative attitude toward self.

Body Boundaries

Throughout the literature, there is a general agreement that the
pregnant woman views her body as a protective container for her fetus
(Deutsch, 1945; Edwards, 1969; Fisher, 1973b; Gray, 1977; McConnell
& Daston, 1961; Rubin, 1970) yet also manifests fears regarding body
intactness and harm (Deutsch, 1945; Edwards, 1969; Fisher, 1973b;
Gillman, 1968; McConnell & Daston, 1961; Plotsky & Shereshefsky,
1969; Rubin, 1970). This view implies that there is a perceptual body
boundary that articulates between the individual and the environment. The body boundary may be defined as the perceived zone of
separation between self and nonself (Fawcett, 1978) that extends
beyond the mere overt physical limitations of one's skin (Fawcett &
Frye, 1980; Fisher & Cleveland, 1968; Horowitz, Duff, & Stratton,
1964). Nearby space and that which occupies the space are integral
parts of one's body boundary (Fisher, 1973a; Fisher & Cleveland,
1968; Schilder, 1970). Two approaches have been taken to study body
boundaries in pregnancy. One approach assesses the degree to which
the body boundary is projected to be either an effective barrier or a
penetrable margin (Fisher & Cleveland, 1968). The other approach
assesses body boundary by determining the amount of body space an
individual perceives the body to occupy (Fawcett, 1977, 1978).

Body Barrier and Penetration. Much of the research in the area of body
boundary has stemmed from the work of Fisher and Cleveland (1955,
1968). In an early research project, Fisher and Cleveland (1955) found

that they were able to categorize responses to inkblot cards according to two separate categories, body barrier and body penetration. Based on this initial work, Fisher and Cleveland (1968) developed barrier and penetration scoring protocols for inkblot responses, which were modified later in 1970 (Fisher, 1970).

Body barrier relates to the protective nature of a boundary, the definiteness of structure, and the surface and substance of quality of the boundary peripheries of an individual (Fisher & Cleveland, 1968). Inkblot responses that are categorized as representing barriers refer to clothing; buildings and enclosed structures; vehicles with holding or containing qualities; concealments, covers, and containers; all living things; all creatures possessing a protective structure; and geographic or natural fomations with delimiting qualities.

Body penetration refers to the boundary's lack of substance, its weakness or fragility, and the ease of entry into it by other objects (Fisher & Cleveland, 1968). Responses to inkblots that are categorized as representing penetration include references to disruption, penetration, damage, or destruction; body openings or acts involving body openings; perceptions involving bypassing or evading the usual boundaries of the body or objects; natural contexts that involve intake or expulsion; and images that are vague or insubstantial in their delimitations.

Barrier and penetration scores are obtained by counting the total number of responses that fall into each of the categories. When a response has both barrier and penetration qualities, the response is counted under both categories. The higher the barrier score, the more protective the body boundary. The higher the penetration score, the less definite the body boundary.

Pregnancy is associated with alterations in body boundaries, as determined by barrier and penetration scores. McConnell and Daston (1961), obtaining barrier and penetration scores on 24 multiparous women in their eighth and ninth months of pregnancy and during the postpartum period, found an increase in penetration scores during pregnancy, followed by a decrease in the postpartum period. Edwards (1969) found a decline in barrier scores for 53 primiparous women during pregnancy and the early postpartum period. Fisher (1973b) also reported that barrier scores declined significantly from the pregnant to the nonpregnant state. Edwards (1969) and Fisher (1973b) did not find that the barrier scores were elevated during pregnancy in comparison to similar samples of nonpregnant women. The fact that barrier scores significantly decreased in the postpartum period and thus were lower than scores for nonpregnant women suggests that there is a change in how the woman perceives her body as a boundary after parturition. Edwards (1969) suggested that the decline in barrier score in the postpartum period might indicate that the woman no longer views her body as a protective container after the baby is born.

Karmel (1975), studying 32 pregnant women of varying parity during the third trimester and six weeks postpartum, plus 28 nonpregnant controls, reported that the pregnant group demonstrated a decline in penetration scores after delivery, while barrier scores were stable throughout the study for both groups. Studying body boundaries with respect to anxiety in 96 primiparous women divided into four groups based on the three trimesters and a postpartum status, Gray (1977) found that (1) barrier scores were lower in the first trimester and the postpartum period than in the second and third trimesters; (2) trait anxiety levels were positively correlated with penetration scores; (3) the mean penetration scores of the subjects was higher than expected, based on Fisher and Cleveland (1968); and (4) there were no significant differences in penetration scores based on trimesters or the postpartum period.

Examination of the findings reported in these body-boundary studies reveals some conflicting results. For example, Edwards (1969) found that barrier scores decreased during pregnancy while Gray (1977) noted a decrease in barrier scores in the first trimester but an increase in barrier scores in the second and third trimesters. The conflicting results may be due to the fact that the samples differed in parity and gestational characteristics. Additionally, the differences found may be due to qualities inherent in the barrier and penetration variables of body boundary. Specifically, some researchers suggest that the barrier variable is not as sensitive to changes, is more stable, and perhaps representative of a personality trait; conversely, the penetration variable behaves more like a state and is thus more sensitive to changes in body boundary (Fisher & Cleveland, 1968; McConnell & Daston, 1961). One notes that, during the postpartum period, barrier scores reported declined significantly from the antepartal period (Fisher, 1973b). This latter finding would suggest that the barrier score may be sensitive to marked physical changes such as those encountered after delivery.

Despite the specific differences in the research findings, two overriding patterns depicting the body boundary do emerge: (1) although the pregnant woman views her body as a protective container, her perception of the body boundary as penetrable and vulnerable to harm is heightened and (2) postpartally, the woman no longer perceives her body as either a special protective container or vulnerable to harm.

Gray's (1977) findings that barrier scores increased in the second and third trimesters directly lend strong support to the claim that the pregnant woman views her body as a protective container. Furthermore, findings by Edwards (1969) and Fisher (1973b) that the barrier score declined significantly from the pregnant to the postpartum state, despite the fact that barrier scores were not elevated above previously established norms for nonpregnant women, also lends some support to the claim that the pregnant woman views her body as a protective container, yet also vulnerable to harm. Penetration scores reported by McConnell and Daston (1961) indirectly indicate that the pregnant body is a protective container and directly indicate that during pregnancy the woman's perception of the body boundary as penetrable and vulnerable to harm is heightened.

Findings reported by Edwards (1969) and Fisher (1973b) also support the claim that after delivery the woman no longer views the body as a protective container. Specifically, in these two studies, barrier scores decreased from the prenatal to the postpartum period. One may speculate that the labor and delivery process itself and the experiences commonly encountered by a woman (i.e., involuntary loss of urine or fecal material, loss of amniotic fluid, expulsion of the baby and the placenta) contribute to the woman's perception that her body is no longer a protective barrier. At the same time, following the delivery, the woman's body is no longer vulnerable to harm. The decreased penetration scores found for postpartum women by McConnell and Daston (1961) and Karmel (1975) lend support to this latter conclusion.

Body Space. Schilder (1970) claimed that the body image is not confined to the body but spreads out into space. Fisher (1973a) noted that individuals perceive the space near their bodies as belonging to them. Body space, a body-boundary perception, is defined as the amount of space an individual occupies, both physically and perceptually (Fawcett, 1976). Thus, an individual's body space includes not only her or his physical body but also nearby objects and space (Fisher, 1973a; Schilder, 1970).

One particular instrument that attempts to measure perception of body space was originated by Schlacter (1971) and modified by Fawcett (1976). This modified topographic device is a 54-inch square of vinyl covered with concentric circles, each circle one inch larger than the preceding one and identified by a two-digit random number (Fawcett, 1976). To assess perception of body space, subjects are asked to stand in the center of the device and to indicate which circle represents the amount of space their bodies occupy. Fawcett (1976) states that subjects are told to imagine that they are encased in a cylinder whose base is one of the circles. The code number of the circle is recorded and converted into inches. Raw scores are reported in inches.

According to the body-image literature, one would hypothesize that the perception of body space would change during pregnancy. This hypothesis is based on three different levels of abstract thought:

1. Body space, by definition, includes one's body, that is, one's actual physical limitation. Accordingly, a change in one's body size should be reflected by a change in body space.
2. The body space acts as a buffer to keep the individual at a safe and comfortable distance from the environment. Thus, as the body size increases in pregnancy, the body space should increase so that a safe and comfortable distance between self and the environment may be maintained.
3. The size of the body buffer zone, or body space, is dependent upon the degree of danger in a situation (Fisher, 1973a). The pregnant woman fears disruption of her body as a result of the impending delivery (Deutsch, 1945). Accordingly, as the pregnancy progresses the body space theoretically increases to protect the woman and her growing fetus.

Fawcett (1976), using the topographic device, demonstrated that both pregnant women and their spouses experienced changes in perception of body space. Specifically, Fawcett found that women and their spouses demonstrated an increase in the amount of perceived body space during the pregnancy, follwed by a decrease during the postpartum period. However, the women perceived a slight rise in perception of body space during the second month postpartum. Fawcett suggests that this latter finding may be due to the fact that in the first postpartum month women felt smaller than they actually were, but, by the second postpartum month, they were aware that they were not as small as they would like to be. In effect Fawcett is pointing out that perception of body space is a reflection not merely of the actual body size but also of an integrative process in which the body's boundary is evaluated physically, psychologically, and socially.

Schuzman (1980) also found that perception of body space is not necessarily reflective of actual body size. Using the topographic device, as modified by Fawcett (1976), to measure body space, Schuzman (1980) compared perception of body space and body size in two groups of pregnant women.The first was called a "descrepancy group" and was composed of 19 women with a uterine size that was small relative to their stage of pregnancy. The second was called a "consistency group" and composed of 19 women with a uterine size appropriate for their dates. Although women in the descrepancy group tended to score high in perception of body space while women in the consistency group tended to score low, the differences were small. Schuzman pointed out that the results may have been influenced by the subjects' self-evaluation of uterine size. Only 6 of the 19 women in the descrepancy group evaluated themselves to have a small uterus. Furthermore, there were 6 women from the consistency group who evaluated their uterus to be small in size for their dates. Of the 12 women who evaluated their uterus as small in size for their dates, those from the consistency group tended to have a small body space,whereas those from the descrepancy group did not demonstrate a pattern. One might suspect from Schuzman's findings that the pregnant woman's self-evaluation of uterine size is a better indicator of body space rather than actual uterine size.

Labor and Delivery: Body-Boundary Experiences. The body boundary changes throughout the pregnancy; however, as labor and delivery approach, the woman frequently experiences anxiety and fears regarding body-boundary intactness and integrity (Angeli, 1978; Bibring et al., 1961; Gillman, 1968; McConnell & Daston, 1961; Plotsky & Shereshefsky, 1969; Tanner, 1969). As the woman undergoes labor and delivery, she may actually experience a loss of body integrity and intactness (Angeli, 1978; Fisher, 1973b; Plotsky & Shereshefsky, 1969; Rubin, 1968) with a concurrent loss of self (Angeli, 1978; Fisher,

1973b). In other words, the laboring woman may experience a body-image disturbance.

Review of the literature reveals that body-boundary disturbances during labor and delivery may arise from internal and external body stimuli. Analysis of case studies reveals that women experience threats to body-boundary integrity through the involuntary loss of bodily contents (Angeli, 1978; Fisher, 1973b;) such as amniotic fluid, urine, blood, stool, and the baby. Furthermore, pain and pressure experienced during the labor and delivery process threaten body-boundary integrity (Fisher, 1973b; Plotsky & Shereshefsky, 1969). The loss of bodily contents and the experience of pain and pressure are accompanied by a feeling that one is no longer in control of one's body. Analgesia and anesthesia may exacerbate the body-image disturbance, while breathing and relaxation techniques may enhance the woman's sense of having bodily control.

Loss of body-boundary integrity may also result from intrusive procedures. Fisher's (1973b) analysis of 37 case studies revealed that the body boundary is threatened by the frequency with which the laboring woman must allow her genitals to be exposed and her vagina and rectum manipulated by fingers or instruments. Fisher also found that being placed in the lithotomy position with a number of strangers present makes the woman feel vulnerable. Based on the literature concerning intrusive procedures and instrumentation, one may hypothesize that, whenever the pregnant woman is subjected to frequent invasive procedures or instrumentation, she may experience a body-image disturbance. Particularly at risk for this would be women labeled as having a high-risk pregnancy, since they frequently must undergo intrusive procedures such as amniocentesis, ultrasound, blood work, fetal monitoring, amnioscopy, and so forth.

Summary

The majority of the literature reviewed indicates that the pregnant woman is aware of the multiple body changes that occur during her pregnancy and may experience a heightened awareness of her body and body parts. Specific body parts may become markedly distorted if the woman experiences conflicts concerning that body part. Marked body-image distortions may also occur if the woman somaticizes the body part. In addition, differences in findings between black and white women suggest that cultural differences may play a part in body awareness and body distortion during pregnancy.

Body boundaries, which include physical and perceptual body space and body barrier and penetration, were found to change throughout pregnancy and during the postpartum period. The literature supports the claim that the pregnant woman views her body as a protective container that is vulnerable to harm. After delivery the woman views her body boundary as less protective, well as less vulnerable.

THE ATTITUDINAL/AFFECTIVE DOMAIN

Individuals have feelings and emotions toward their own bodies and those of others. People's body images are, in part, manifestations of these feelings and emotions toward their own bodies as well as reflections of their perceptions of how others feel about their bodies. The *attitudinal domain* of body image refers to those feelings and emotional reactions toward the body (Fawcett, 1978). In essence, the attitudinal domain of body image is an affective domain representing intrapersonal and interpersonal values. Similarly, during pregnancy, the woman's attitudes toward her body reflect her personal appraisal of the multiple body changes and how she compares to nonpregnant and other pregnant women, as well as the evaluation of her pregnant body by significant others and the society at large.

Body Attitude Assessment Tools

Two tools, primarily, have been used to assess the pregnant woman's attitudes toward the pregnant body: the Body-Cathexis Self-Cathexis Scale (Second & Jourard, 1953) and Osgood's Semantic Differential (Osgood, Suci, & Tannenbaum, 1975). Both tools have been used in modified versions.

Body-Cathexis Self-Cathexis. The original, unadapted Body-Cathexis Self-Cathexis tool (Secord & Jourard, 1953) consists of 40 body-cathexis and 40 self-cathexis items which subjects rate on a 5-point scale, with 1 indicating a strong positive feeling and 5 indicating a strong negative feeling. A raw score is obtained by adding the respective scores of answers for each of the items.

The majority of the research using the Body-Cathexis Self-Cathexis Scale has eliminated the Self-Cathexis times, the Body-Cathexis Scale is believed to represent an individual's degree of satisfaction with the body, but even the Body-Cathexis Scale is not always used in its complete form. Most often researchers select which items to test. As a result, the strength of the findings and the ability of a particular piece of research to support or refute other findings is questionable. The original tool has a split half reliability range of $r = .78$ to $r = .83$ (Secord & Jourard, 1953).

Osgood Semantic Differential. Osgood's Semantic Differential (Osgood et al., 1975) measures attitudes toward the body. The tool is based on the premise that an attitude is learned, is potentially bipolar, and can be identified through semantic dimensions. Three major dimensions of attitude are measured: evaluation, potency, and activity. The tool consisits of several paired adjectives (e.g., potency: tough–fragile; evaluation: beautiful–ugly; and activity: active–passive). Subjects are asked to evaluate a person (e.g., self, husband, wife, ideal woman, ideal man) in terms of the bipolar adjectives on a Likert scale. A semantic profile emerges. A score is obtained whereby a high score is more negative. The original tool has a test-retest reliability of .87 to .93 (Osgood, 1952; Snide & Osgood, 1969). However, as with the other attitudinal scale, researchers have selected different items to test, thus diminishing the ability to generalize and fully compare the results.

Attitudes toward the Pregnant Body

As the pregnancy progresses, the woman's appraisal of her body changes. Initially most women welcome the overt proof of their pregnancy, proudly displaying their pregnant state. As Moore (1978) noted, pregnancy is the ultimate proof of femininity. Yet, as the pregnancy advances, the uterus/abdomen greatly enlarge; the breasts become heavy; the thighs, buttocks, and shoulders increase in bulk, and weight gain seems unlimited. Women now often harbor negative feelings about their bodies (Tannner, 1969). In particular Tanner found that women focused upon their enlarging abdomens as the source of their feeling awkward and unattractive. Using scores on the Body-Cathexis questionnaire to compare 20 pregnant women in the third trimester with 20 nonpregnant women, Ruggieri et al. (1979) found that pregnant women held significantly more negative feelings about their bodies than nonpregnant women. Moore (1978), using the Osgood Semantic Differential, demonstrated that pregnant women view themselves as less attractive than usual and less attractive than the ideal woman. Furthermore, pregnant women consider themselves as uglier, more awful, having a more annoying body, dirtier, heavier, larger, older, and slower than usual and/or than the ideal woman (Moore, 1978). Testing husbands, Moore found that men did not react as strongly to their wives' bodies but did see their wives as being weaker, more tense, fatter, and larger. Moore (1978), like Tanner (1969), found that the adjectives *larger* and *fatter* often were applied to the increased abdominal size and weight noted in the pregnant woman.

The studies by Tanner (1969), Ruggieri et al. (1979), and Moore (1978) all lead to the same conclusion that, as the pregnancy progresses, the woman harbors negative attitudes. Moore's (1978) study also leads one to believe that the pregnant woman's level of satisfaction with her body is determined by cultural/social norms and by significant others' appraisals of the pregnant body.

Schuzman (1980) hypothesized that pregnant women who did not meet the culturally determined norms for uterine/abdominal size would be more dissatisfied with their bodies than women with uterine/abdominal sizes that were normal for their dates. Schuzman's scores on the Body-Cathexis Scale for 19 women with a uterine-size/date discrepancy, compared with 19 women with uterine-size/date consistency, did not support this hypothesis. However, she did find that women who perceived that the father of the baby or a significant other female thought that the uterus was normal in size were more satisfied with their bodies. These findings suggest that pregnant women place greater importance on the appraisals of their bodies by significant others than they do on the medical evaluation. In addition, in contrast with the original expectation, Schuzman found that women who evaluated their own uteruses as small in size demonstrated a high degree of satisfaction with the body. One may speculate that these women were more satisfied with their bodies because the perceived smaller uterine/abdominal size is more consistent with the ideal female figure as well as with their own usual nonpregnant state. Unfortunately, the Body-Cathexis Scale does not distinguish between those women who are satisfied or dissatisfied with their bodies because their bodies do or do not meet expectations for body size during pregnancy; nor does it distinguish those who are satisfied or dissatisfied with their bodies because their bodies do or do not meet the ideal, socially accepted, and valued body image. In this respect, Osgood's Semantic Differential may shed more light on women's satisfaction with the body during pregnancy.

Body Attitudes and Anxiety

The decreased satisfaction with the body may be accompanied by an increase in anxiety. Testing 138 primigravidas, Gordon (1976) found a significant inverse relationship between level of anxiety and expressed satisfaction with the body as measured by the Body-Cathexis Scale. Gordon did not find a corresponding higher incidence of maladaptive physiological responses, as one might expect with increased anxiety. One might expect, however, that if anxiety rose to a high level, the pregnant woman might manifest both physiological and psychological maladaptive behaviors. Such behaviors preclude the woman from successfully completing the tasks of pregnancy (Budd, 1977).

Personality Traits and Body Attitudes

The pregnant woman's attitude toward her body may also reflect personality characteristics. Three pieces of research lend support to this statement. McConnell and Daston (1961) found that pregnant women with positive attitiudes tended to have higher barrier scores and lower penetration scores than pregnant women with negative attitudes. Furthermore, the pregnant women with positive attitudes tended to evaluate their bodies positively during the pregnancy but negatively afterward; whereas pregnant women with negative attitudes during the pregnancy evaluated their bodies positively afterward. The researchers speculated that the pregnant women with positive attitudes placed importance on the ability of their bodies to protect and contain their babies. In contrast, they suggest that pregnant women with negative attitudes may feel as if their bodies have been penetrated by a foreign object.

Venezia (1972) did not find a significant relationship between body attitude and attitude toward pregnancy, but did find relationships between body attitude and the personality variables of introversion-extroversion. Specifically, Venezia (1972) reported that extroverted women evaluated their bodies more negatively during the third trimester than introverted women.

Lastly, Sherwen (1983) evaluated the effect of the psychoprophylactic method (PPM) of childbirth preparation on body attitudes with respect to women's perception of locus of control (i.e., the degree to which an individual perceives a causal relationship between her own behavior and a reinforcement). Sherwen (1983) reported that, after receiving PPM, women who reported internal locus of control experienced an increase in body cathexis compared to women reporting external locus of control.

The findings of McConnell and Daston (1961), Venezia (1972), and Sherwen (1983) strongly suggest that preexisting personality traits are reflected in the pregnant woman's body attitude.

Summary

In the first trimester of pregnancy a woman generally has a positive body attitude; however, as the pregnancy advances and the physical body is most discontinuous with the usual body configuration and sensations, the woman's body image becomes more negative. The attitude the woman holds toward her pregnant body also reflects her previously held beliefs and personality traits. Women who value their ability to conceive and maintain a pregnancy may have a more positive attitude during pregnancy. Furthermore, women who tend to focus on internal stimuli as opposed to external stimuli may have a greater propensity for a positive body attitude during pregnancy.

SIGNIFICANCE OF BODY IMAGE IN PREGNANCY

Pregnancy is a developmental process that has as its ultimate goal the establishment of a foundation for the mother-infant relationship and the woman's upcoming role of mother. Theoretically, the rapidly occurring somatic and psychological changes of pregnancy create psychological upheaval and turmoil requiring the pregnant woman to master specific psychological tasks (Budd, 1977; Tanner, 1969). There are five main psychological tasks of pregnancy:

1. Working through the idea of being pregnant
2. Adjusting the body image.
3. Viewing the fetus as a separate object.

4. Readiness and preparation for labor and delivery and anatomical separation from the fetus
5. Readiness and preparation for the caretaking or maternal role

The pregnant woman completes these psychological tasks through observable behaviors (Tanner, 1969). Adjustment of the body image is an ongoing task dealt with by the pregnant woman (Budd, 1977; Tanner, 1969) and is a corequisite for the completion of third-trimester tasks.

The first antepartal event of conception creates physical and psychological changes necessitating the woman's body image to augment and incorporate the embryo/fetus as an extension of self. The second antepartal event of quickening, at about 20 weeks of gestation, is accredited as being the major stimulus for viewing the fetus as a separate being (Bibring et al., 1961; Rubin, 1970; Tanner, 1969). Viewing the fetus as a separate being allows the woman to prepare for the caretaking role and physical separation. It is unlikely, however, that fetal movement, present from the twentieth week of gestation, is the only stimulus for completing the tasks that remain. The overt and profound changes in the outward form and appearance of the body and how the woman feels about these changes are implicated in the completion of the tasks. More specifically, the negative feelings about one's body in the third trimester lead to a disenchantment with the pregnant state (Colman & Colman, 1971; Rubin, 1970; Tanner, 1969). The woman now wants the pregnancy to end. Essentially, the disenchantment with the pregnant body expressed in the third trimester should stimulate the woman to tackle overtly the tasks that prepare her for labor and delivery, anatomical separation from the fetus, and motherhood.

NURSING IMPLICATIONS

Nurses are in the position to promote the development of a healthy body image in pregnancy. The phrase, *healthy body image,* is used here to mean a realistic view of one's body, its changes, and the implications of those body changes. The literature reviewed indicates that body image does change during pregnancy and the postpartum period. Generally, a pregnant woman experiences a change in body size, shape, configuration, body boundaries, body space, and body satisfaction.

Specific body parts become focused upon (e.g. abdomen/uterus) and may be distorted, while overall body awareness and body distortion may not be significantly different from the nonpregnant state. In general, pregnant women do not experience a body-image disturbance; rather, they appropriately integrate body changes into their body image. Failure to augment the body image during pregnancy may interfere with laying down the foundation for motherhood. In addition, body-image disturbances resulting from the labor and delivery experience may physically and emotionally immobilize the woman, thus delaying the taking on of the maternal role (Angeli, 1978; Rubin, 1970).

Nursing Assessment

Nursing assessment of the pregnant woman's body image should be carried out at each prenatal visit, during labor and delivery and the initial postpartum period, and at the postpartum follow-up. This schedule is recommended so that body-image problems can be detected as early as possible and interventions initiated.

Body image can be assessed easily through interviews with the pregnant woman. The nurse assesses what changes, if any, the woman has perceived in her body and how the woman feels about these changes. Sample questions are given in Table 7-1. Although the woman's self-perceptions and attitudes toward her body may be personality bound, perceptions and attitudes of the pregnant body should generally fall within the norms for a given culture. For example, the degree of satisfaction with the body should be more positive in the first and second trimesters than in the third trimester. Women who manifest perceptions and attitudes that greatly differ from the norms may be demon-

Table 7-1. Sample Interview Questions for Body-Image Assessment

What changes have you noticed in your body?
What changes did you expect in your body?
Describe how you think you look now.
When you think of how you look, how do you feel emotionally?
What does a significant other tell you about your body?
Do you agree with significant others' opinions about your body?
How do you think you appear to others?

strating either a personality difference or a body-image disturbance. Through interviews, the nurse can determine the meaning of the woman's perceptions and attitudes.

Body image in pregnant women may be observed in part through specific behaviors (e.g., validating the pregnancy, wearing maternity clothes, and telling others about the pregnancy). Since augmentation of the body image is an ongoing process and is corequisite for task work during pregnancy, the successful completion of the tasks of pregnancy is indicative of appropriate body image augmentation during pregnancy. Table 7-2 lists the five tasks of pregnancy, discussed previously, along with emotions and behaviors that should be associated with each which would indicate good progress.

During labor and delivery, the nurse must frequently rely on nonverbal cues to the woman's body image perception and attitude. Women who are having difficult labors requiring instrumentation, augmentation, or medication, as well as those needing a Cesarean section, may express a negative body attitude.

During the initial postpartum period, the nurse should reassess the woman's body image and attitudes concerning the labor and delivery experience. The postpartum woman may need help integrating her labor and delivery experience into her body image. Frequently, the woman needs to verbalize what she experienced and how she felt. Furthermore, women who had difficult labors may feel inadequate. They also may feel as if their bodies were assaulted.

In addition to interviewing the woman in the postpartum period, the nurse can assess the body image through observing behaviors. How the woman interacts with others, in particular the baby and the father of the baby, may reflect whether the woman is integrating the labor and delivery experience into her body image. Failure to interact with the newborn, failure to initiate any caretaking behaviors after a couple of days, or expressed anger or indifference toward the baby or father of the baby may be clues that the woman is feeling negatively about herself.

Nursing Intervention

Nurses need to provide information concerning expected physical changes of pregnancy and their psychological counterparts. Women should be helped to evaluate the changes they are undergoing or have undergone and to incorporate these changes successfully into their

Table 7-2. The Five Tasks of Pregnancy, with Associated Behaviors and Emotions

1. Augmenting the Body Image (all trimesters)
   Integrates changes in body image through all subsequent tasks

2. Working through the idea of being pregnant (first trimester)
   Validates pregnancy
   Ambivalence changes to acceptance of pregnancy
   Seeks information about physical changes
   Tells significant others about pregnancy
   Views fetus as extension of self

3. Recognizes the fetus as a separate being (second trimester)
   Quickening detected by woman
   Views fetus as separate being
   Fantasizes of infant of 4-5 months of age
   Wants a vision of the baby
   Has others feel fetal movement
   Wears maternity clothes
   Begins purchase or makes plans for baby items
   Tells others of pregnancy
   No longer ambivalent

4. & 5. Readiness for labor and delivery and anatomical separation from the fetus; readiness for the caretaking and maternal role (third trimester)
   Focuses on enlarged abdomen
   Describes self as awkward and unattractive
   Disenchanted with pregnant state, but not with fetus
   Body image most discontinuous with usual state
   Numerous fantasies about the baby in terms of sex, size, appearance
   Baby names tried out
   Visualizes a newborn
   Handles baby items
   Decides on method of feeding baby
   Nesting behaviors
   Prefers to stay at home

---

body image. Nurses need to help women anticipate the possible changes and to plan on the means for dealing with them. All pregnant women should be educated about common procedures and instruments used during pregnancy, labor and delivery, and the postpartum period. The information provided about procedures and instruments should include the sounds and sensations women experience during and after the experience. These measures may prevent body anxiety and a body-image disturbance. Before, during, and after such procedures the nurse needs to provide reinforcement of the information given, as well as supportive measures.

Women who experience difficulty during procedures, have a difficult labor, or have a Cesarean section may need additional help in integrating the experience. The nurse needs to encourage the woman to verbalize her feelings and to view the experience realistically, so that positive aspects of the experience do not get overshadowed by the negative aspects.

When working with a woman with a body-image disturbance, the nurse needs to determine first the extent and severity of the disturbance. Minor body-image disturbances may be handled through problem-identification and problem-solving techniques; however, women who manifest extreme disturbances (e.g., denial of pregnancy) need psychiatric evaluation and follow-up. In these extreme situations referrals need to be made.

REFERENCES

Angeli, D. (1978). Body boundaries: Concerns of a laboring woman. *Maternal-Child Nursing Journal, 7,* 41–46.

Bibring, G., Dwyer, T., Huntington, D., & Valenstein, A. (1961). A study of psychological processes in pregnancy and of the earliest mother-child relationship. *Psychoanalytic Study of the Child, 16,* 9–71.

Budd, K. (1977). Behavioral tasks of the high-risk maternity patient. In N.A. Lytle (Ed.), *Nursing of Women in an Age of Liberation.* Iowa: W. C. Brown.

Caplan, G. (1961). The psychology of pregnancy and the origins of mother-child relationships. In Caplan, G. (Ed.), *Approach to community mental health.* New York: Grune & Stratton.

Colman, A., & Colman, L. (1971). *Pregnancy: The psychological experience.* New York: Herder & Herder.

Corbreil, M. (1971). Nursing process for a patient with a body image disturbance. *Nursing Clinics of North America, 6,* 155–163.

Demspey, M. (1972). The development of body image in the adolescent. *Nursing Clinics of North America, 6,* 155–163.

Deutsch, H. (1945). *The psychology of women* (Vol. 2). New York: Grune & Stratton.

Edwards, K. (1969). *Psychological changes associated with pregnancy and obstetric complications.* Doctoral dissertation, University of Miami, Miami, Florida.

Fawcett, J. (1976). *The relationship between spouses' strength of identification and their patterns of change in perceived body space and articulation of body concept during and after pregnancy.* Doctoral dissertation, New York University, New York, NY.

Fawcett, J. (1977). The relationship between identification and patterns of change in spouses' body images during and after pregnancy. *International Journal of Students, 14,* 199–213.

Fawcett, J. (1978, July/August). Body image and the pregnant couple. *Maternal Child Nursing,* pp. 227–233.

Fawcett, J., & Frye, S. (1980). An exploratory study of body image dimensionality. *Nursing Research, 29,* 324–327.

Fisher, S. (1970). *Body experience in fantasy and behavior.* Norwalk, CT: Appleton-Century-Crofts.

Fisher, S. (1973a). *Body consciousness: You are what you feel.* Englewood Cliffs, NJ: Prentice-Hall.

Fisher, S. (1973b). *The female orgasm: Psychology, physiology, fantasy.* New York: Basic Books.

Fisher, S., & Cleveland, S. (1955). The role of body image in psychosomatic symptom of choice. *Psychological Monographs: General and Applied, 402,* 1–15.

Fisher, S., & Cleveland, S. (1968). *Body image and personality.* New York: Dover Press.

Gillman, R. (1968). The dreams of pregnant women and maternal adaptation. *American Journal of Orthopsychiatry, 38,* 688–692.

Gordon, S. (1976). *Relationships among anxiety, expressed satisfaction with body image and maladaptive physiological responses in pregnancy.* Unpublished doctoral dissertation, New York University, New York, NY.

Gray, L. (1977). *A study of pregnancy: Body image and anxiety.* Doctoral dissertation, California School of Professional Psychology, Los Angeles.

Harris, R. (1979). Cultural differences in body perception during pregnancy. *British Journal of Medical Psychology, 52,* 347–352.

Horowitz, M., Duff., D., & Stratton, L. (1964). Body buffer zone: Exploration of personal space. *Archives of General Psychiatry, 11,* 651–656.

Karmel, R. (1975). Body image characteristics of late pregnancy and changes observed at the postnatal period. In H. Hirst (Ed.), *The family. 4th International Congress of Psychosomatic Obstetrics and Gynecology.* Tel Aviv, Israel: Karger Basel.

Kolb, L. (1959). Disturbances of the body image. In S. Arieti (Ed.), *American handbook of psychiatry.* New York: Basic Books, 749–769.

Leonard, B. J. (1972). Body image changes in chronic illness. *Nursing Clinics of North America, 7,* 687–695.

McConnell, O., & Daston, P. (1961). Body image changes in pregnancy. *Journal of Projective Techniques, 25,* 452–456.

Moore, D. (1978). The body image in pregnancy. *Journal of Nurse-Midwifery, 70,* 502–508.

Murray, R. (1972). Body image development in adulthood. *Nursing clinics of North America, 7,* 617–630.

Norris, C. (1978). Body image: Its relevance to professional nursing. In C. Carlson & B. Blackwell (Eds.), *Behavioral concepts and nursing intervention.* Philadelphia: Lippincott.

Osgood, C. (1952). The nature and measurement of meaning. *Psychological Bulletin, 49,* 197–237.

Osgood, C., Suci, L., & Tannenbaum, R. (1975). *The measurement of meaning.* Urbana, IL: University of Illinois Press.

Petrella, J. (1978, July/August). The unwed pregnant adolescent. *Journal of Obstetrical and Gynecological Nursing,* pp. 22–26.

Plotsky, H., & Shereshefsky, P. (1969). The psychological meaning of watching the delivery. *Child and Family, 8,* (Summer) 254–264.

Rubin, R. (1968, June). Body image and self esteem. *Nursing Outlook,* pp. 20–23.

Rubin, R. (1970). Cognitive style in pregnancy. *American Journal of Nursing, 70,* 502–508.

Ruggieri, V., Milizia, M., & Romano, M. (1979). Effects of body image on tactile sensitivity to a tickle: A study of pregnancy. *Perceptual and Motor Skills, 49,* 555–563.

Schilder, P. (1970). *The image and apprearance of the human body.* New York: International Press.

Schlacter, L. (1971). *The relation between anxiety, perceived body and personal space among young female adults.* Unpublished doctoral dissertation, New York University, New York, NY.

Secord, P. (1953). Objectification of word association procedures by the use of homonyms: A measure of body cathexis. *Journal of Personality, 2,* 479–495.

Secord, P., & Jourard, S. (1953). Body cathexis and the ideal female figure. *Journal of Social Psychology. 50,* 243–246.

Sherwen, L. (1983). An investigation into the effects of psychoprophylactic method training and locus of control on fantasy production and body cathexis in the primiparous woman. In L. N. Sherwen & C. T. Weingarten (Eds.), *Analysis and application of nursing research: Parent-neonate studies.* Monterey, CA: Wadsworth Health Sciences Division.

Schuzman, E. (1980). *Body image with respect to completion of psychological tasks of pregnancy.* Masters thesis, Case Western Reserve University, Cleveland, Ohio.

Snide, J., & Osgood, C. (1969). *Semantic differential technique.* Chicago: Aldine.

Tanner, L. (1969). Developmental tasks of pregnancy. In B. Bergersen, E. Anderson, M. Duffey, M. Lohr, & H. Rose (Eds.), *Current concepts in clinical nursing.* St. Louis: C. V. Mosby.

Tolar, A., & Digrazia, P. (1977). The body image of pregnant women as reflected in their human figure drawings. *Journal of Clinical Psychiatry, 33,* 566–571.

Uddenberg, N., & Hakansan, M. (1972). Aniseikonic body perception in pregnancy. *Journal of Psychosomatic Research, 16,* 179–184.

Venezia, D. (1972). *Correlates of body attitude change in pregnancy.* Doctoral dissertation, Washington University, St. Louis, MO.

Weinberg, J. (1978). Body image disturbance as a factor in the crisis situation of pregnancy: A review. *Journal of Obstetrical and Gynecological Nursing, 7,* 18–21.

Chapter 8

The Pregnant Man

Only recently have health care providers considered the father of importance during childbearing and childrearing. The majority of research and theoretical literature concerning the father and his role in pregnancy and in relation with the child has been produced in the last 10 years. Much remains unknown in this area. Studies concerning the father, especially during pregnancy, are basically descriptive in nature. Much that is known comes from case studies, psychoanalytic analyses of fathers in treatment, and the clinical experience of practitioners.

Several content areas in the literature shed some light on the state of the father during his mate's pregnancy and on the changes he must undergo as the entire family system alters. These areas include

1. *Evolution of the role of father.* The fathering role seems to evolve in three distinct and interdependent ways: through developmental factors inherent in the father and situational factors inherent in the family system and its environment; through a man's participation in the childbearing cycle; and through the father-infant interaction.
2. *Paternal experience of pregnancy.* This experience includes both physical, bodily perceptions (the couvade syndrome, with its symptomology) and psychological perceptions (paternal fantasies).

These areas, as they concern the father during the phase of family-system pregnancy, will be explored. Suggestions for interventions with the father as part of the pregnant family will be made.

EVOLUTION OF THE FATHERING ROLE

Developmental and Situational Aspects

The evolution of the fathering role can be viewed from a developmental framework. It is seen to begin in childhood and evolves as part of normal childhood growth and development. Ross (1982) has traced the psychoanalytic literature to uncover the "roots" of fatherhood. In general, it seems to indicate that both girls and boys go through various phases where they wish to create and give birth to babies. In addition, boys identify with their mothers, and thus their nature contains many "maternal" elements. Gradually, the boys' wishes and attitudes concerning childbearing are transformed into more traditional patterns of fathering, generally through interaction and identification with their fathers. However, a boy's (and eventually, a man's) urge to create life remains linked to what the psychoanalysts call "maternal ambitions." Kestenberg, Marcus, Sossin, and Stevenson (1982) reinforce the concept of a man's paternal attitudes being rooted in dual identifications with mother and father. These attitudes contain both maternal (nurturant) aspects and paternal (provider-protector) aspects, the latter often exaggerated. They further state that, to become truly paternal or maternal, individuals of each sex must borrow certain characteristics from the other. The borrowing is, then, the essence of their bisexuality and is a prerequisite for successful parenting.

In a present-oriented approach, Cronenwett and Kunst-Wilson (1981) offer a stress framework for understanding paternal role transition. The paradigm implicates such factors, said to affect paternal role evolution, as individual or situational conditioning variables, objective stress (such as objective role conflict), perceived stress (such as subjective role conflict), and coping and defense responses of the father. The interaction of all such variables, specific to the father's unique situation, will determine both short-term responses to evolution of the paternal role (as anxiety or depression) and enduring outcomes (as paternal role attainment and fulfillment).

Soule, Stanley, and Copans (1979) surveyed 70 first-time prospective fathers, aged 20 to 42 years, during the last month of their wives' pregnancies, to ascertain the factors associated with development of "father identity." While concluding that expectant fathers vary widely in their abilities to picture themselves in the paternal role, they were able to identify some factors that correlated highly with a strong, positive paternal identity. These investigators found that income was negatively correlated to father identity (FI), while marital satisfaction and haste to conceive a child were positively correlated. Father identity (FI) also reinforced and was reinfored by emotionally positive pregnancies. Liking children was not a significant source of fatherly feelings, but men who had extensive experience with infants seemed to be fathering enthusiasts. Finally, a man's relationship as a child with his own father seemed especially important in this study, although current parental support seemed to be negatively related to development of a positive FI. Pleasant memories of being fathered or lingering dissatisfaction with the relationship may impel a man either to repeat or more successfully rework his past in his own fathering role.

It becomes clear from this brief discussion on evolution of the paternal role that such role transition is a developing function that draws from and influences many areas of life experience. Fathering is a complex interweaving of the biological, cultural, and intrapsychic aspects of the man.

Participation in the Childbearing Cycle

Several authors and investigators indicate that the father's active participation in the pregnancy and delivery will assist with the evolution of the paternal role (in his wife's and his own eyes) and in his attachment to the newborn. Colman and Colman (1971) felt that men who participated in their wives' childbirth were given the means for coping with the intense feelings associated with the birth. Chabon (1966) also stated that participation in the psychoprophylactic method (PPM) of childbirth preparation permits the father to have an active, supportive role in the childbirth.

Tanzer and Block (1976) reported that women whose husbands had been with them during labor and delivery described their husbands in positive terms, while women whose husbands were not with them described their husbands in negative terms. Goodwin (1970) also reported a great difference between PPM and nonPPM women in descriptions of husbands. PPM women, who had their husbands with them in labor and delivery, gave highly positive accounts of their husbands and their performances during labor and delivery.

Porter and Demeuth (1979) found that a husband's involvement in the planning of a pregnancy affects his acceptance of that pregnancy.

Hott (1980), in comparing two groups of PPM-prepared mothers and fathers (those who were able to share labor and delivery, versus those who were not due to complications necessitating a cesarean delivery) found that fathers prevented from participating in the delivery tended to see themselves as less active. Bowen and Miller (1980) examined the relationship between paternal presence at prenatal classes and delivery, and the father's infant-attachment behaviors. They found that father presence at delivery emerged as an important variable related to observable attachment behaviors of fathers to their newborn infants.

Active involvement in pregnancy, labor, and delivery seems to make a difference not only in the man's perception of himself as a father but also in the mother's perception. Further, participation in the childbearing cycle seems to be important in the evolving father-infant relationship.

Father-Infant Interaction

Greenberg and Morris's (1974) classical study, which uncovered the phenomenon of paternal "engrossment" in the newborn, made it evident to future researchers that the infant plays an important role in the father-infant relationship and assumption of "fathering" or the paternal role. The literature contains many studies that indicate the importance of father-infant interactions to bond formation and role evolution in the father. Further studies investigate effects of interventions planned to enhance paternal-newborn interactions.

Parke has been active in attacking what he calls "myths" concerning fatherhood (Parke, 1975; Parke, Power, & Fisher, 1980). In a review of studies and in his own and his associates' investigations concerning fathering, Parke concludes that fathers are interested and involved in their newborns, that they can be nurturant and can assume caretaking roles relative to the newborn, and that fathers can be as competent as mothers in care of newborn infants.

Kotelchuck (1972), Pedersen and Robson (1969), and Earls (1977), in a variety of observational studies, concluded that both paternal and maternal bonds are dependent on the amount of interacting and caretaking given by the parent to the infant. Paternal attachment was specifically associated with the amount of caretaking, strength of emotional investment, and amount of stimulating play the father involved himself in with the infant. Parke, in addition, stressed the function of play in establishing the father-infant relationship and the role of father (Parke, 1975).

Chibucos and Kali (1981) in a study of 19 father-infant dyads, found that quality of the father-infant interaction at two months of infant age predicted the security of infant-father attachment at 7½ months. Frodi (1980), after an extensive review of the literature on fathering, concluded that there is no support for a hormonal explanation of female preparedness to be more sensitive to newborns. She suggested that sensitivity to the newborn is a consequence, rather than a cause, of involvement with infants.

Studies designed to facilitate father-infant bond formation and hence movement into the paternal role have implicated the role of caretaker and also the function of teaching the father caretaking skills. Bills (1980) studied effects of planned physical contact on enhancement of paternal-newborn bond formation. In a comparison of 15 fathers who had planned contact that included teaching the fathers skills in handling the infant, and a control group of 15 fathers who did not have such contact, Bills demonstrated that physical contact expedited the acquaintance process and enhanced the paternal–newborn affectional bonds.

Wandersman (1980) studied 47 first-time fathers by means of self-reports of their feelings of well-being, sense of competence as a parent, views of their babies' temperaments, marital relationships, and social support systems. Self-reports were recorded at 2 to 3 months, 5 to 6 months, and 9 to 10 months after birth. Wandersman concluded that quality of the marital relationship and attendance at parenting groups (N = 20 fathers) were associated with positive adjustment to the baby at 9 to 10 months and to the paternal role.

Taubenheim (1981), in a descriptive study of first-time fathers, attempted to document the process of paternal-infant bonding. Her primary finding was that fathers who fed their infants had the most "bonding behaviors," as measured by an observational tool. She concluded that engaging in caretaking behaviors may be an important element in the process of paternal–infant attachment and may facilitate paternal role assumption.

Finally, Bloom-Feshbach, Bloom-Feshbach, and Gaughran (1980), after exploring the relationship of three-year-olds' separation distress and parental childcare styles, concluded that it is more appropriate to conceptualize parental functions than maternal and paternal roles.

Findings of this study suggest the necessity of the interchangeability of parenting functions. Flexibility in allocation of childcare responsibilities is seen as particularly important in light of contemporary changes in sex roles.

Conclusions

From the material presented in this section on evolution of the paternal role, several conclusions can be drawn concerning fathering. First, a man is, to some extent, developmentally programmed to be a father. Such "fathering" is composed of nurturing and instrumental (provider/protector) components, evolved through identification with mother and father, respectively. The socialization process and the father's unique circumstances will help to determine the exact manifestation of the paternal role in a man.

Second, a man's active involvement throughout childbearing seems to assist with evolution of the paternal role. This is true not only from the father's perspective but also from the mother's. In addition, the father's presence at the delivery seems to initiate a positive father-newborn interaction.

Finally, the literature supports the notion that fathers can be as nurturant of children as can mothers. Father-newborn interaction helps to usher in this nurturing involvement as part of the paternal role. Further, planned intervention to increase paternal–newborn contact and teach the father caretaking skills seems to facilitate this process.

It becomes evident, then, that fathers are often involved and highly interested in pregnancy, infants, and their paternal role evolution.

THE FATHER'S EXPERIENCES DURING PREGNANCY

Benedek (1970) saw the roots of fatherhood lying in a man's instinctual drive for survival (biological fulfillment) and in the potential it holds for further evolution of his personality. In each culture, the prospective father undergoes specific changes designed to help him assume his role. These changes are often prescribed by a culturally dependent ritual.

Bodily Perceptions: The Couvade

Each culture has a system of ceremonies and rituals that provide its culture carriers with a universe that is orderly and understandable. As Aamodt (1978) indicates, ritual behaviors provide the means for the reenactment of the relationships among the symbolic elements in the cultural system and allow for the incorporation of the sense of the meaning of these symbolic elements into the daily lives of individuals in that culture.

Ceremonies and rituals associated with childbearing have been developed in most societies, focusing on life-cycle events, including childbirth. Rules or prescriptions for the roles of mother and father vary among cultural systems. For example, many cultures prescribe that fathers be isolated from the processes and activities of pregnancy, birth, and puerperium. Another type of ritual, however, encourages men to participate in the birth of their offspring. This ritual is the couvade, practiced by some South American Tribes. In this ritual, the husband, in a setting separated from his parturient wife, mimics the childbearing process of his mate. At the same time his wife indicates the onset of labor and retreats to the care of selected women in the community, the husband goes to a hammock and proceeds to go through the motions of childbirth. This practice, according to the culture practicing it, attracts evil power to the husband, thus luring it from the mother and ensuring the safe delivery of the newborn (Aamodt, 1978).

Although the dominant culture of the United States does not hold such specific beliefs, it recently has begun to encourage men to participate more intimately in the childbearing cycle. This "couvade ritual" involves classes for childbearing in which fathers are trained and prompted to take part in pregnancy, labor, delivery, and care of the newborn. In addition, men involved in childbearing experience psychological changes that many practitioners and theoreticians liken to the couvade ritual seen in the more primitive cultures. Colman (1969) saw the function of the couvade ritual in the United States as allowing the father to play a role during pregnancy and childbirth. This perception of couvade would assist him to evolve into the role of father and gain acknowledgment from his mate and society. It further would help him to cope with envy of and competition with his mate's creative reproductive function.

A variety of descriptive studies or surveys have identified a father's involvement with pregnancy and have extended our knowledge regarding couvade symptoms. Liebenberg's (1969) study found fathers expressed envy of the pregnancy either by fusing with the wife in an attempt to experience the pregnancy in a biological sense, or by denying the pregnancy. He further noted development of pregnancy symptoms in 65% of his pregnant fathers. Indications of paternal pregnancy symptomology also come from Trethowan and Conlon (1965) and from Trethowan (1968). Using retrospective and longitudinal designs, these investigators found that British men experienced symptoms of physical illness during their mates' pregnancies, including gastrointestinal disorders, increased or decreased appetite, backache, and toothache. In interviews of American men, Munroe and Munroe (1971) found reports of sympathetic symptoms of pregnancy including nausea and vomiting, syncope, lassitude, leg cramps, weight gain, and backache, during the period of the wife's pregnancy. In his 1969 study, Liebenberg further observed paternal concerns concerning body intactness in husbands of pregnant women. Such findings of paternal symptomology are confirmed cross-culturally (Munroe & Munroe, 1971; Munroe, Munroe, & Nerlove, 1973).

Trethowan and Conlon (1965) coined the term *couvade syndrome* to describe these paternal bodily symptoms during pregnancy. Couvade phenomena are said to be an expression of a prospective father's involvement in pregnancy and his identification with his mate (Colman & Colman, 1971; Trethowan, 1968). Colman and Colman (1971) further believed that a husband's close proximity to his wife influenced his response to the pregnancy. The more he identified with her, the greater would he experience changes in his body during the pregnancy. Fawcett (1977) attempted to confirm a link between paternal identification with pregnancy and change in body space perception during pregnancy, but was unable to do so. She did note, however, that perceived body space of husbands changed during and after the wives' pregnancies, although the form and appearance of the men's bodies did not change.

Psychological Processes of Pregnancy

In addition to couvade symptoms and perceived bodily changes during pregnancy, prospective fathers may be aware of other psychological changes. These psychological changes begin to usher in paternal role taking and prepare the man for parenting an infant. Some of the most vivid descriptions of psychological changes during pregnancy, including many fantasies, come from case studies of individuals undergoing psychoanalysis (Gurwitt, 1982). Herzog (1982) also reports on a retrospective study of pregnancy experiences of 103 first-time fathers whose wives had given birth prematurely. In combination with the case study descriptions, such information can give some insight into the psychological pregnancy experiences of men.

Herzog (1982) was able to categorize the 103 men involved in his study into two distinct groups: those who were in touch with feelings and fantasies pertaining to the pregnancy, and those who were not (he further divided the fathers who were not in touch with feelings and fantasies into his "less" and "least" attuned groups). Herzog felt that men who were cognizant of their own feelings concerning the impending arrival of their first child were also empathic with and invested in their wives. Further, since men can choose (consciously or unconsciously) to be at least once removed from the actual events of pregnancy, childbirth, and childrearing, psychological participation in the events and experience reflects their previous life experiences, conflicts, and conflict resolution. Herzog, in his reports of common experiences, focused on the experiences of his "highly attuned" father group (N = 35), contrasting them to the experiences of his "less attuned" and "least attuned" father groups.

Herzog (1982) divided the psychological processes of pregnancy for attuned fathers-to-be into the following time periods, based on Gurwitt's (1982) distinctions:

1. *Getting ready.* This was a distinct period, perceived by fathers, in which both mother and father knew they would try to make a child soon. Emotionally, fathers reported a feeling of embarking on something new and foreign. Fathers felt an urgency "to get on with it."

2. *Conception.* This period occurred when the conception was medically confirmed. The affective characteristic of this phase was one of joy. Additionally, fathers-to-be reported a surge of manliness and a heightened interest in sexual behavior with their wives.

3. *End of the first trimester.* Fathers now perceived a great change in their lives, first marked by an increase in new and different fantasies during lovemaking. Contact with themes of expectant fatherhood was achieved in the sexual realm. Fathers reported feelings and images of themselves as nurturing or fertilizing their fetuses, their wives, and the

pregnancy. Feelings of "having to give" and "feeding" the fetus during intercourse were prevalent.

4. *Midpregnancy.* Fathers in the attuned group now often reported gastrointestinal symptoms. In addition, some fathers reported feelings and wishes that they could both "fertilize" and "bear" a child; some felt "empty" inside. Many fathers in this group reported that they began to eat more, and some gained much weight during this phase.

5. *Turn toward own father and fathering role.* Between 15 and 25 weeks, attuned fathers reported an increased pressure to sort out things with their families of origin, especially their relations with their own fathers. One preoccupation was to "reestablish connections" with the past generations. Without this sorting-out phase, men were seen to be less able to participate in expectant fatherhood.

6. *End of pregnancy.* At 26 to 28 weeks, those fathers who experienced the pregnancy as long as the third trimester (remember, these births were all premature) reported feeling that something powerful, magical, and "big"—beyond their ability to control—was going on. Fathers indicated a perceptible shift toward readying things in the real world for the child's arrival. Observations of children, concerns with patterns of childrearing, and preparation for the infant's arrival replaced preoccupations with inner thoughts and processes.

In this study, fathers in the attuned, less attuned, and least attuned groups all had the process of becoming a father cut short by premature deliveries. All fathers reported experiences (in varying degrees) of anger, distress, grief, and fear toward the unexpected aspects of childbirth.

Paternal fantasies during pregnancy are another important psychological process for the father-to-be. Herzog (1982) reported fantasies throughout the aforementioned phases. As discussed, at the end of the first trimester, attuned fathers had sexually oriented fantasies of "feeding" the mother, fetus, and pregnancy during intercourse with the wife. During the phase of turning toward father and fatherhood (#5), attuned fathers reported fantasies of "plumbing, circuitry, and other kinds of connecting" (p. 308). After quickening, fantasies turned to the coming child. The father-to-be, in general, began to think of the fetus as a child, separate from his wife or himself. The sex of the child was now visualized (usually a boy). Blatantly aggressive and intrusive fantasies now made an appearance in the fathers' reports, and fathers became aware of a "wish to hurt the baby as well as to welcome it" (p.

309). Finally, in Herzog's study, toward the end of pregnancy, intrusive fantasies declined, and a shift was made to prepare for the coming child in the real world.

Gurwitt (1982), in his case study of an expectant father, also mentioned dream reports and feelings during pregnancy that are of interest for this chapter. During the getting-ready phase (#1), images and symbols reported by the father reflected themes of birds, nesting, and egg hatching. Night dreams reflected a fear of being "left out" by the pregnancy, and symbols of lakes and shores were recalled. The father described in the study felt a need to "create" himself, in this case by completing a thesis. During the conception phase (#2), dream reports again referred to bodies of water, this time the ocean and shore. The expectant father's thoughts revolved around death and competition with his own father and wife. During the midpregnancy phase (#4), dreams concerned a symbolic representation of a "full uterus" that had no room for the father. Paternal feelings included increased lability and rapidly shifting themes. This father-to-be was now very aware that the pregnancy "involved a baby." In addition, feelings that his wife was "ugly" surfaced. During the final phase of pregnancy (#6), the case-study father felt more positive about the childbirth cycle; his image of his wife shifted to one of her beauty; and he began to work through feelings of jealousy of and competition with his wife and fetus. Dreams again were of water and diving. At the end of the pregnancy, themes of magic and mysticism were prevalent in this father's life and fantasies. Additional dream content was related to the baby coming and the birth process.

While it is impossible to extrapolate from a case study to the general population of pregnant fathers, the reports of this father's feelings and fantasies give some insight into possible aspects of an expectant father's state during pregnancy. Similarities to Herzog's (1982) reports of his attuned fathers' experiences are evident.

Some empirical documentation for this descriptive data comes from Gerzi and Berman (1981). These investigators tested 51 expectant fathers during the last three months of their wives' first pregnancies with an IPAT Anxiety Scale and the Blacky Picture Test, a well-known projective instrument. They compared their results to 51 married men without children, tested on the same instruments. They found significantly higher overall anxiety in the expectant-father group, plus greater oedipal intensity, sibling rivalry, guilt feelings, ambivalence, infantile fantasies, feminine identifications, and castration fears. Such tests seem to give some credence to the previously described reports of paternal experience of pregnancy.

Operating under the assumption that fantasy state during pregnancy may be one indicator of an expectant father's psychological well-being, Sherwen (1986) studied the paternal third-trimester fantasy pattern and its relation to the father's degree of involvement in the pregnancy and his sex-role orientation. The following questions were investigated:

1. Do expectant fathers present a different fantasy pattern than do nonexpectant men?
2. Do expectant fathers present a fantasy pattern similar to expectant women?
3. Does sex-role orientation relate to the expectant father's fantasy pattern?
4. Does paternal involvement in the pregnancy relate to the expectant father's fantasy pattern?

The total volunteer sample consisted of 38 primiparous third-trimester couples enrolled in Lamaze classes and a convenience sample of 40 nonexpectant males. Three instruments were used for the comparisons necessary to answer the research questions: the 10 Scale Imaginal Processes Inventory (IPI), which measures fantasy pattern; the Bem Sex Role Inventory (SRI), which measures sex-role orientation; and the Bills Affectional Relationship Inventory (ARQ), which indicates the extent of paternal involvement in the pregnancy. Expectant parents were asked to record any remembered day and night dreams.

Results demonstrated several significant findings. Of the 10 IPI subscales used in the study, expectant fathers demonstrated a significantly higher score ($p < .04$) on the Present-Oriented Fantasy Subscale than did nonexpectant men. Expectant fathers and mothers presented a similar fantasy pattern, except on the Nightdreaming Frequency Subscale. Mothers had significantly higher scores ($p < .004$) than did fathers. Fathers were divided by the BEM SRI into three groups based on sex-role orientation: feminine (N = 7), masculine (N = 11), and androgynous (N = 20). Significant differences between groups were found on the Fear of Failure Fantasies, Bizarre Improbable Fantasies, Present-Oriented Fantasies, Visual Imagery in Daydreams, and Frightened Reactions in Daydreams subscales, Post-hoc t-tests indicated that fathers with a feminine orientation had significantly higher means on most of the aforementioned scales. Finally, paternal involvement in pregnancy as measured by the ARQ was positively related to Positive Reactions in Daydreams and Visual Imagery in Daydreams. Paternal involvement was inversely related to Daydreaming Frequency and Future-Oriented Daydream subscales.

In addition, Sherwen (1986) was able to group together paternal fantasies based on recurrent themes, in a manner similar to the maternal fantasy categories described in an earlier chapter. Expectant men, in addition to filling out questionnaires, were informally asked to write down any day or night dreams they may have had in the course of the pregnancy. Twenty-seven fathers reported one or more fantasies; 58 fantasy descriptions were obtained in total. Although these data are very tentative, a variety of themes seemed to be reflected in the fantasy descriptions.

The most prevalent theme (30 fantasies) was the father's anxiety with the upcoming events (e.g., being a good father, anxiety over the condition of the wife or infant, having a cesarean delivery, not having enough money). An example of this type of fantasy is

> "They (nightdreams) seem to have originated from fear. In one . . . my wife gave birth to a boy that seemed to be deformed or disfigured."

A second common theme (13 fantasies) was the father's happiness with the coming events:

> "I always have this picture in my mind of coming home from work and being greeted on the front porch by children, wife, and the dog barking happily in the background."

A third theme found in 5 fantasy descriptions was the fear of damage or trauma to the self, spouse, or significant other, such as the wife being mugged or attacked. Another theme (4 fantasies) was the father's winning or coming into large sums of money, such as winning the lottery. Four fantasies also concerned the theme of being prepared:

> "I keep imagining that the baby will arrive and I won't be prepared — no film, not packed for the hospital, the Lamaze bag not ready . . . "

Three fantasy descriptions fell under the theme of loss and/or death:

> "I imagine where my deceased friends have gone to."

Three fathers also described using fantasy to solve problems in work situations. Other fantasy descriptions were on the following topics (one fantasy each): the father's own creativity and/or dependents, such as acquiring and caring for dogs; the reactions of others, especially the father's father, to the child; the father retiring early and having great amounts of leisure time; and having intercourse with a thin woman.

Sherwen (1986) made some tentative conclusions based on her data:

1. There seemed to be some difference in the fantasy pattern of expectant fathers, compared to nonexpectant men, on the fantasy scale of Present-Oriented Daydreams, with expectant fathers having more present-oriented fantasies.
2. Mothers and fathers during pregnancy do not manifest significantly different fantasy patterns, except on the scale of Night-dreaming Frequency. Mothers demonstrated a much higher mean score on this variable, a trend that seemed to parallel earlier findings (Sherwen, 1983).
3. Sex-role orientation may, in some way, affect fantasy pattern in expectant fathers. Whether a father has a masculine, feminine, or androgynous orientation may be one factor that will determine how the father perceives and reacts to his mate's pregnancy.
4. The extent of paternal involvement in the pregnancy also seems to have some relation to the fantasy pattern demonstrated by expectant fathers. These relationships may stimulate much additional investigation.
5. Expectant fathers seem to have recurrent themes in fantasy, as do expectant mothers. These themes may give clues to a father's current concerns.

Another aspect of the father's psychological state during pregnancy discussed by Herzog (1982) and mentioned briefly earlier, is that some men are "attuned" to their inner state and some men are not. This aspect of pregnancy is elaborated on by May (1980), who did an exploratory study of the experiences of 20 first-time expectant fathers in order to generate grounded theory that describes a typology of "styles" adopted by fathers during pregnancy. May's theory explains, in part, the phenomenon of the father's involvement in pregnancy.

Such involvement, according to May, has two polar dimensions: detachment or involvement. These dimensions are interwoven into what this investigator calls the three styles of paternal pregnancy experience:

1. *Observer style.* The man reports a certain emotional distance from the pregnancy and sees himself largely as a bystander. This style is the most detached of the three, involves little decision making in the pregnancy, and can have either a happy or unhappy affective state associated with it.
2. *Expressive style.* The man reports a highly emotional response to pregnancy and sees himself as a full partner in it. This style allows for more involvement in the pregnancy, and often those fathers who adopt this style have a high incidence of pregnancy symptoms. These fathers also expect to parent their children actively.
3. *Instrumental style.* The man reports an emphasis on tasks to be accomplished and sees himself largely as a caretaker or manager of the pregnancy. These fathers downplay the emotional impact of the pregnancy and pride themselves in carrying out traditional functions central to their roles as husbands and fathers. They "take care of business," often making appointments for their wives, keeping their wives on diets, and making major purchases and decisions concerning the infant. Such a style represents a midpoint along the detachment-involvement continuum.

Conclusions

From the studies discussed in this section, it would seem reasonable to state that expectant fathers do perceive changes in their physical and psychological states during a mate's pregnancy, yet without actual physiological alterations. The extent of the changes that are involved in the couvade syndrome and in changes in the psychological state need to be identified, to illuminate better their function in paternal role evolution and in paternal–infant relationships. Brazelton (1982) notes that, among his clients, prospective fathers generally indicate that no one has ever asked them anything about the pregnancy or their role in it. Brazelton asks, "Isn't this too bad at a time when we are expecting them to play a vital role once the baby arrives?" (p. 16).

NURSING INTERVENTION: WORKING WITH THE FATHER-TO-BE

It seems somewhat premature, based on research concerned with fathering, to suggest nursing interventions for work with fathers in the pregnant family system. Even at our present early state of knowledge concening the father-to-be's experience during pregnancy, however, certain broad principles for health care and guidance present themselves. Key to these principles, again, is the concept of the developmental or maturational crisis. The father-to-be must master tasks concerned with becoming a parent and rearing a child. How a man resolves his own developmental crisis will effect the overall efficiency of the family system in mastering its developmental tasks. Interventions can be categorized to fall into "precrisis" and "crisis" stages.

Precrisis State

Anticipatory Guidance. The father-to-be may not even be aware that he will be undergoing changes as part of the evolution of his new role. Preparing him for the new feelings, conflicts, and fantasies he may have during his mate's pregnancy may be a vitual step in facilitating his adoption of the fathering role. In addition, it may also be that a father-to-be has had minimal experience with pregnant women and with infants. Preparing him for possible changes in his mate, the events of labor and delivery, and the characteristics and care of newborns will most likely be important forms of anticipatory guidance.

Assessment of Strengths and Weaknesses (risk factors). A knowledge of a father-to-be's role in his family of origin; his past exposure to children and crisis situations; his cultural views of masculinity, femininity, and parenting; and his desire to be or not to be involved in the pregnancy are some factors that can give clues to the ease with which a man may make the transformation to fatherhood. For example, a man who has cared for children and infants in his family of origin would generally have a definite strength in entering into the role of father. On the other hand, a man who has a deeply ingrained cultural prohibition against a man's involvement in pregnancy and nurturing will have a real conflict in assuming an active involvement with childbearing. This is not to say that all adequate fathers must take an active role in the pregnancy and in nurturing the newborn. A father-to-be needs to identify a style of fathering that is comfortable to him and acceptable to his mate. Cultivating guilt over a father's inability to be active during pregnancy is not in the best of interests of family evolution.

Identification of Resources. Part of precrisis intervention for the father-to-be may be identification of support systems and resources, both within and outside of the family system. The father may need to identify sources of financial aid to assist with the cost of childbearing. He may need external interests and challenges to allow him to develop his own creative needs. He may need to redefine and reevaluate relations with his family of origin, especially his own father; and he may need to identify sources, both professional and personal, where he can get emotional support as he "fuels" his wife's system.

Crisis State

Assessment and Planning Intervention. During the perinatal period, the father (as well as the mother) needs to have certain needs met if he is to function adequately in the family. The nurse must accurately assess the father's "style" of fathering before actually planning interventions. This might be done through observing the extent of detachment and involvement in the pregnancy, according to May's (1980) classifications (the observer, expressive, and instrumental styles).

Active Intervention. Once the nurse has ascertained the father's appropriate level of involvement in the birthing process (his style), appropriate experiences may be devised to meet his needs. Before the birth, active involvement in childbirth preparation classes is fairly common for fathers. Depending on the father's inner awareness and desire to be involved in pregnancy, these classes might be expanded to include imagery exercises, which will allow the father further participation in and understanding of the birth. Classes may also include physical exercises that the father who is experiencing couvade symptomology might do with his mate.

During labor and delivery, the father should be allowed to seek his own level of involvement, without being made to feel guilty. The nurse should be available to support both mother and father during the experience. If desired, both the father and mother can bond with the newborn immediately after birth, allowing the father to begin his engrossment with his child. All through the prenatal period, the father who desires such involvement can learn infant caretaking skills. After delivery, both father and mother can be taught (and teach each other) such caretaking skills as infant bathing and the use of infant stimulation techniques.

Future Planning. The nurse may assist the new family in defining a structure for caring for their new child. Reorganization of family space and time, realignment of roles and responsibilities, and relating to other children in the family are all aspects of future planning that will help cement family function on a higher level.

In parting, it should be emphasized that the preceding suggestions are still tentative in nature. Nurses and health care providers have traditionally ignored the father throughout the course of his mate's pregnancy, therefore, there are few interventions designed specifically to facilitate paternal adaptation to pregnancy and the paternal role. In addition, there is little research documenting effects of various intervention strategies on these variables. Work with and research into the state of the father during pregnancy should be a nursing priority. Evolution of "good" fathers is as important as evolution of "good" mothers when considering the family as a whole.

REFERENCES

Aamodt, A. Culture. (1978). In A. Clark (Ed.), *Culture child-bearing health professionals.* Philadelphia: F. A. Davis.

Benedek, T. (1970). Fatherhood and providing. In E. J. Anthony and T. Benedek (Eds.), *Parenthood.* Boston: Little, Brown.

Bills, B. J. (1980). Enhancement of paternal-newborn affectional bonds. *Journal of Nurse-Midwifery, 25*(5), 21–25.

Bloom-Feshbach, S., Bloom-Feshbach, J., & Gaughran, J. (1980). The child's tie to both parents: Separation patterns and nursery school adjustment. *American Journal of Orthopsychiatry, 50*(3), 505–521.

Bowen, S. M., & Miller, B. C. (1980). Paternal attachment behavior as related to presence at delivery and preparenthood classes: A pilot study. *Nursing Research, 29*(5), 307–311.

Brazelton, T. B. (1982). Comment. In M. Klaus & J. Kennel (Eds.), *Parent-infant bonding.* St. Louis: C. V. Mosby.

Chabon, I. (1966). *Awake and aware: Participating in childbirth through psychoprophlaxis.* New York: Delacorte Press.

Chibucos, T. R., & Kail, P. R. (1981). Longitudinal examinations of father-infant interaction and infant-father attachment. *Merrill-Palmer Quarterly, 27*(2), 81–96.

Colman, A. (1969). Psychological state during first pregnancy. *American Journal of Orthopsychiatry, 39,* 788–797.

Colman, A., & Colman, L. (1971). *Pregnancy: The psychological experience.* New York: Herder and Herder.

Cronenwett, L., & Knunst-Wilson, W. (1981). Stress, social support, and the transition to fatherhood. *Nurisng Research, 30*(4), 196–201.

Earls, F. (1977). The fathers (not mothers): Their importance and influence with infants and young children. In S. Chess & A. Thomas, (Eds.), *Annual Progress in Child Psychiatry and Child Development,* Tenth Annual Edition. New York: Brunner/Mazel.

Fawcett, J. (1977). The relationship between identification and patterns of change in spouses' body images during and after pregnancy. *International Journal of Nursing Studies, 14,* 199–213.

Frodi, A. M. (1980). Paternal-baby responsiveness and involvement. *Infant Mental Health Journal, 1*(3), 150–160.

Gerzi, S., & Berman, E. (1981). Emotional reactions of expectant fathers to their wives' first pregnancy. *British Journal of Medical Psychology, 54*(3), 259–265.

Goodwin, B. (1970). *An investigation of the relationships between psychoprophylaxis in childbirth and changes in concept of self and concept of husband.* Unpublished Doctoral Dissertation, New York University, New York, NY.

Greenburg, M., & Morris, N. (1974). Engrossment: The newborn's impact on the father. *American Journal of Orthopsychiatry, 44,* 521.

Gurwitt, A. R. (1982). Aspects of prospective fatherhood. In S. Cath, N. Gurwitt, & J. M. Ross (Eds.), *Father and child.* Boston: Little, Brown.

Herzog, J. M. (1982). Patterns of expectant fatherhood: A study of the fathers of a group of premature infants. In S. Cath, N. Gurwitt, & J. M. Ross (Eds.), *Father and child.* Boston: Little, Brown.

Hott, J. R. (1980). Best laid plans: Pre and postpartum comparisons of self and spouse in primiparous Lamaze couples who share delivery and those who do not. *Nursing Research, 29*(5), 307–311.

Kestenberg, J., Marcus, H., Sossin, K., & Stevenson, R. (1982). The development of paternal attitudes. In S. Cath, N. Gurwitt, & J. M. Ross (Eds.), *Father and child.* Boston: Little, Brown.

Kotelchuck, M. (1972). *The nature of the child's tie to his father.* Unpublished Doctoral Dissertation, Harvard University, Cambridge, MA.

Liebenberg, B. (1969). Expected fathers. *Child and family, 8,* 265–278.

May, K. A. (1980). A typology of detachment/involvement styles adopted during pregnancy by first-time fathers. *Western Journal of Nursing Research, 2*(2), 445–453.

Munroe, R. L. & Munroe, R. H. (1971). Male pregnancy symptoms and cross-sex identity in three societies. *Journal of Social Psychology, 84,* 11–25.

Munroe, R. L., Munroe, R. H., & Nerlove, S. B. (1973). Male pregnancy symptoms and cross-sex identity: Two replications. *Journal of Social Psychology, 89,* 147–148.

Parke, R. D. (1975). The father's role in infancy: A re-evaluation. *Birth and the Family Journal, 5*(4), 211–213.

Parke, R. D., Power, T. G., & Fisher, T. (1980). The adolescent father's impact on the mother and child. *Journal of Social Issues, 36*(1) 88–106.

Pedersen, R. A., & Robson, K. S. (1969). Father participation in infancy. *American Journal of Orthopsychiatry, 19,* 466–472.

Porter, L., & Demeuth, B. (1979). The impact of marital adjustment on pregnancy acceptance. *MCN, The Maternal-Child Nursing Journal, 8* (1), 103–112.

Ross, J. M. (1982). In search of fathering: A review. In S. Cath, N. N. Gurwitt, & J. M. Ross (Eds.), *Father and child.* Boston: Little, Brown.

Sherwen, L. (1983). An investigation into the effects of locus of control and psychoprophylactic method training on body cathexis and fantasy production in the primiparous woman. In L. Sherwen and C. Weingarten (Eds.), *Analysis and application of nursing research: Parent-neonate studies.* Monterey, CA: Wadsworth.

Sherwen, L. (in press). Third trimester fantasies of first time expectant fathers. *MCN, The Maternal-Child Nursing Journal.*

Soule, B., Stanley, K. & Copans, S. (1979). Father identity. *Psychiatry, 42*(3), 255–263.

Tanzer, D., & Block, J. (1976). *Why natural childbirth?* New York: Shocket Books.

Taubenheim, A. M. (1981). Paternal-infant bonding in the first-time father. *Journal of Obstetric, Gynecological and Neonatal Nursing, 10,* 261–264.

Trethowan, W. H. (1968). The couvade syndrome—Some further observations. *Journal of Psychosomatic Research, 12,* 107–115.

Trethowan, W. H., & Conlon, M. F. (1965). The couvade syndrome. *British Journal of Psychology, 3,* 57–60.

Wandersman, L. P. (1980). The adjustment of fathers to their first baby: The roles of parenting groups and marital relationship. *Birth and the Family Journal, 7*(3), 155–161.

Chapter 9

Responses of Siblings to Pregnancy

Susan Kutzner

Families represent complex social systems that comprise a network of relationships (Zigler, Lamb, & Child, 1982). These family networks are critical to understanding family dynamics and, more important, individual development. The problem that arises for health professionals and researchers is to determine how interactions among family members affect the psychological and social development of individuals, especially children. One basic assumption that has been made in the past is that family interactions are associated with group and individual responses and personality development.

More recent research has focused on individual perceptions of specific events related to reproductive and psychosocial issues in family life. Researchers in nursing such as Mercer (1981, 1983, 1986a & b), Rubin (1985), and others have described the mother's perception of her role. The interpretation of a mother's perception of her role helps to delineate the family's health and the family's adaptation to a particular developmental phase of a child, parent, or the familial unit as a whole.

This chapter focuses on sibling relationships as a dynamic force within the family, which may or may not be associated with personality development, family psychological health, and parent-child interactions. In nursing and developmental psychology, researchers now utilize interactional theory (Lamb, Suomi, & Stephenson, 1979) to change the perspective of research from parental effects on children to one of children's effects on parents, with an emphasis on the mutual influences that children and parents exert upon each other. Initial studies by Lamb (1976, 1977, 1978, 1979) focused on the effects on the parent's presence on the interaction between an infant and its other parent, within an interactional model. Mercer (1981) utilized a theoretical framework that outlined attainment of the maternal role. The mother's perceptions of her infant and other children were measured at six points during the first year after birth of a child. Other studies by Lederman, Lederman, Work, and McCann (1979), Sherwen (1980), Kutzner (1984), Weingarten (1985), and others, through longitudinal research designs, have alluded to the interactional processes within families.

Critical questions may be posed regarding the psychosocial responses of siblings to pregnancy as a critical family milestone. While the literature has indirectly described the relationships children have with each other via parental and others' perceptions, few studies are focused on the siblings' responses to a critical reproductive event in the family. This chapter focuses on related literature that helps to elucidate pregnancy and postpartum issues. Sibling responses to pregnancy, birth, and the postpartum period will be described as well as parental responses to the siblings' adjustment during these periods. Finally, implications for nursing practice and research will be presented.

LITERATURE REVIEW

Developmental Themes

Families are composed of networks of relationships that can involve parents, siblings, grandparents, and others in the extended family. Currently, clinicians and researchers are questioning how the interactions of family members, specifically siblings, affect their development and adaptation. Dunn (1983) describes two themes in developmental psychological research that suggest that sibling relationships may have developmental implications. The first theme emphasizes sibling differences in regard to personality, intellectual development, and psychopathology, "although they share not only more genetic material than unrelated children but many aspects of the family environment" (Scarr & Grajek, quoted in Dunn, 1983, p. 789). Differences between siblings may be explained by their direct influence on each other, the differences in specific parent–child interactions, and the differing aspects of the family environment. Dunn (1983) speculates that siblings create different environments for one another through their interactions with each other.

The second theme reflects the current thought among researchers that a focus on the mother and child as a dyad isolated from the family unit is quite misleading. Bronfenbrenner (1979), Clarke-Stewart (1978), Lamb (1976), Lewis and Rosenblum (1979), and Parke, Power, and Gottman (1979) have demonstrated the complexity of interactional processes within the family. Dunn (1983) suggests that "it seems highly likely that the relationship between young siblings will affect and be affected by the children's relationship with their parents" (p. 787).

Certainly, the maternal–child nursing research in the past 10 years reflects a holistic approach to the study of families. Mercer's (1981, 1983, 1986a,1986b) current papers demonstrate a preliminary "untangling" of the various components of maternal perceptions surrounding a reproductive experience such as childbirth and the early years of child development. A comparison was made between adolescent mothers and older mothers: "Although age groups . . . (15–19 years, 20–29 years, and 30–42 years) . . . functioned at different levels, their patterns of behaviors over the years did not vary, except for gratification in the role, indicating that the maternal role presented similar challenges for all women" (1986a, p. 205). Mercer's work suggests that a child's developmental phase has an effect on the perceptions of the mother and her role: "The departure from a positive linear increase in maternal attainment behaviors was a discontinuity for which the women appeared unprepared, yet the developing child continues to present different challenges throughout childhood and adolescence" (1986a, p.12).

Although it is possible to speculate about the effect of the child on the mother, few studies have been designed to assess social interaction factors. Bronfenbrenner (1974, 1975, 1976, 1977) suggests that many developmentally significant effects might be mediated indirectly through another person rather than through direct interaction with the child. This issue is important because it indicates the necessity of studying indirect as well as direct effects of children and parents upon one another. Lamb (1979) is concerned "with effects on the immediate *interaction* rather than with long-term effects on the child's personality" (p. 255) and is interested in a descriptive approach to the complexity of family interactions, rather than a focus on predictive modeling of future child behavior. This longitudinal approach within a social interaction model also provides a series of data that demonstrates patterns and trends in parent and child behaviors and development. Kutzner (1984), Lederman (1979), Mercer (1981), Weingarten (1985), and others have studied mothers, fathers, and children from this perspective. Although their theoretical frameworks differ somewhat, the studies utilize similar samples and background literature and have comparable results.

Overall, these studies of mothers, fathers, and their children (including sibling relationships) focus on the influence of several key variables, as defined by Sameroff (1975): the continuum of reproductive casualty (high risk factors which might affect later development), anoxia, prematurity, newborn status, and socioeconomic influences. Of these variables, "socio-economic status appears to have much stronger influence on the course of development than perinatal history" (Sameroff, 1975, p. 292). Infants from lower-class homes showed significant deficits three to five years postpartum, in comparison to infants from upper-class homes with identical histories of perinatal complications. Moreover, there are higher rates of prematurity and low-birth-weight babies in areas of low socioeconomic status and poor access to health care in metropolitan areas.

Sameroff (1975) proposes a "continuum of caretaking causality," which includes environmental risk factors leading toward poor developmental outcomes in children. The factors include deficiencies in interactional patterns among family members, such as in parent-child, child-parent, and sibling relationships. Sameroff and Chandler (1975) suggest that some characteristics of children may predispose them to be victims of child abuse. For instance, an association was found between low birth weight and battered child syndrome (Klein & Stern, 1971). Klaus and Kennel (1970), and Weingarten (1985) speculate that a premature infant may stress mothers and fathers who have limited resources and who create poor adaptation patterns. Kutzner (1984) finds that mothers who perceive their labors and deliveries as difficult and/or negative experiences associate those feelings with their child three to four years after delivery.

While cases of obvious pathologies in parenting can be identified with developmental problems in children, it is difficult to assess the effects of child-caretaker relations (Sameroff, 1975). The literature reviewed by Sameroff supports "the hypothesis that knowing *only* the temperament of the child or knowing *only* the child-rearing attitudes and practices of parents would not allow one to predict the developmental outcome for the child. It would appear, rather, that it is the character of the *specific transactions* that occurred between a given child and his parents which determined the course of his subsequent development" (pp. 8-9).

Sibling Studies Overview

There are over 2,000 documented studies on birth order of children which have directed interpretations and speculations about siblings of varying ages. Wagner, Schubert, and Schubert (1975), in a review of these studies, find that the last century's research deals with primogeniture only; that is, the studies contrast firstborn children with only children. Major sibling variables from these studies include sibship size, ordinal position, and sibling age spacing. The dependent variables are intelligence, achievement, creativity, personality, and health. Wagner et al. feel that there are predictable and investigatable issues in birth order. Even if one focuses on the sibship variables, however, the studies have evolved to include improved research designs and better articulation of complex variables. For example, Koch (1954) limited study families to those with two children and assessed the effects of spacing. Sibling dyads were identified as older males with younger males, older females with younger males, and vice versa.

One pattern that emerges from studies of sibship size is that the larger the family, the lower the mean intelligence quotient (IQ). Zajonc and Markus (1975) find an association between a large family size and low academic achievement. Cicirelli (1977), however, in another related study, finds that, due to confounding with family size, birth order should not be used to explain children's achievement without considering other sibling-structure variables. It may be speculated that, within a large group of individuals, a decreased level of language may be evident among the younger siblings due to their being raised by children instead of adults.

Most of this research involves middle-class samples. Cross-lag studies have been conducted utilizing path analysis (e.g. Clarke-

Stewart 1978; and others). While one cannot infer causality, there was a significant relationship between scores on The Bayley (1969) Scales of Infant Development at 11 months and maternal attitude at 17 months. Studies focusing on the effects of sibship and personality traits have found that different maladjustments are present in smaller families as compared with larger families.

The health care professional or researcher must exercise caution when interpreting these studies. The exact variables are not clearly articulated; thus it is difficult to interpret one group as differing from another. The data focus predominantly on middle-class samples, excluding the lower and upper socioeconomic groups. It is possible that the findings of low IQ or academic achievement in large families are not present if the large family has sufficient economic resources and time to spend with children, or no economic resources or time to spend with any of the children.

The effects of ordinal position of each sibling can be pervasive in a child's development. A sibling's position in the family can influence social relationships and possibly relationships with other siblings. For instance, some studies have found that if there is time to devote to the parent–child relationship with the first child, the child may influence the parents' relationship to each other and to later children (Dunn, 1983; Kutzner, 1984). Age spacing is a critical variable. Researchers have observed that two closely spaced children are treated alike, often to the detriment of the older child (Bryant, 1982; Cicirelli, 1982; Schachter, 1982). The parents and older sibling speak at the level of the younger child and play games at the level of the younger child. When the children are widely spaced, it is easier for the parents to meet the needs of each individual child.

Sex of the sibling has been studied; some results show that the sex of the oldest child affects the welcome of the next child (Dunn, 1981).

Finally, the only child is subject to certain myths in the United States, such as beliefs that the only child can be selfish, arrogant, and unsharing. However, only children are under- and over-represented in certain groups, a finding that belies these myths. These children are rarely found in groups with high rates of juvenile delinquency. They are overrepresented among scientists and scholars. Many social scientists are among only children but are rarely seen as politicians or lawyers. Female only children are overrepresented among actresses, especially if the parents are separated (Falbo, 1982). Other literature has led researchers to generalize personality traits in only children

(Blake, 1981; Claudy, Farrell, & Dayton, 1979). Overall, these children are felt to be adult-oriented, socially rigid, and more trusting than other children with siblings. The males and females are thought to show more feminine characteristics, most likely due to the increased time with their mothers.

SIBLING AND PARENTAL RESPONSES
TO PREGNANCY, BIRTH, AND THE POSTPARTUM PERIOD

Recently there has been a greater emphasis in sibling research on interactions within families. Most studies have assessed birth order and other variables without focusing on the quality of interaction between children or on important developmental milestones in families, such as reproductive events. Eighty percent of all children in the United States and Europe grow up with siblings (Dunn 1985). The relationships between siblings and parents provide clues for understanding the development of young children and new parents. To date, observational research has provided data about frequency of interactions, the interest of siblings in one another, how siblings imitate behavior, and evidence of teaching and attachment. Dunn (1985) suggests "sibling interaction may influence not only the nature of the later relationship between children but also the personality of each sibling as an individual" (p. 797).

Longitudinal studies by Dunn and Kendrick (1982a) and Lamb (1978) show patterns of influence by firstborn children and later-born children toward each other. These studies suggest that the pattern of individual differences in the sibling relationship are established during the infancy of the secondborn child and continued throughout early childhood (Dunn, 1985).

There are few descriptions of children's reactions to the birth of a sibling. The public in general and professional writers as well often allude to negative sibling behaviors during pregnancy and the postpartum months. There are clinical reports of sibling responses such as being upset, sleep disturbances, frequent crying, regressive behaviors (especially in regard to toilet training), demanding negative behavior, and so forth. At the same time, Dunn (1985) points out that "the presence of the new baby is not only a source of disturbance—it is of very great interest to most firstborn children" (p. 9).

Dunn and Kendrick (1979, 1980) observed that the arrival of a sibling was associated with changes in interactional patterns between firstborn children and their mothers. Mothers spent less time with their firstborn children while attending to the needs of the newborn. Also, an increase in confrontation and maternal restraint was noted (Dunn & Kendrick, 1980). Kendrick and Dunn (1980) studied the direct effects of the mother's attention to the new baby on interaction between the mother and first child. The sample consisted of 40 families, interviewed and observed at two time points: one to three months before the expected date of delivery of the second child and two to three weeks postpartum. Sex differences were not significant. There was, however, an increase in both confrontation and positive involvement between the mother and firstborn child. In contexts where the mother was not involved with the new infant, there was still a decrease in maternal attention after the sibling birth.

Nadelman and Begun (1982) demonstrated that sibling influences begin even before the child is born, for the anticipation of the expected birth affects the parents as well as their relationships with and their availability to their firstborn offspring. Corter, Abramovitch, and Pepler (1983) described sibling interaction in relationship to maternal role. They found that maternal presence was related to a reduction in overall level of sibling interaction; sibling interaction also tended to be relatively more "agonistic" when the mother was present than when she was absent.

Most current studies, however, have not focused on the effect of sibling interaction on the maternal role. Maternal adaptation may be influenced by the developmental phases of each child in the family, as well as by the sibling relationship itself. The mother's anticipation of the effects of her children upon her attainment of her motherhood role and the realities of mothering tasks are interesting issues to consider, as they provide information (via maternal perceptions) on family functioning. In a preliminary study of 36 mothers and fathers, Kutzner (1984) observed patterns among parents that indicated the sibling relationships as perceived by the parents portrayed mirror images of their marital relationships. Parents mentioned that their own experiences as siblings in their families influenced how they wanted their children to relate to each other. Many mothers also equated positive views of their children's relationships with their confidence in themselves. Finally, mothers and fathers compared their children's relationships with those of their friends and other relatives. The parents frequently mentioned how alike or different their children's relationships were from their friends' children; they perceived success or failure in their children's relationships as a direct measure of their success as parents.

Contemporary sibling research is beginning to provide clues as to the effects siblings have on each other and their parents, especially with the emphasis of current work on developmental phases of children, new parents, and interaction theory. Pregnancy, childbirth, and the postpartum period are all significant familial developmental phases. These phases have become increasingly complex because of new parental responsibilities and activities. Contemporary factors include working parents, increasing dependence on daycare, and societal and economic changes. Professionals in nursing and other health fields encourage the preparation of firstborn children and other siblings for the birth of a new child; however, currently available research has not provided an adequate assessment of the theoretical premises for these programs. For some children, involvement in prenatal classes for and the delivery of their siblings, as well as immediate postpartum visits, help to alleviate anxiety due to maternal separation. Yet there are no data demonstrating a decrease in regressive and other antagonistic behaviors as the newborn infant matures.

In addition, there is no evidence to indicate that parents are supported in the early phases of childrearing with anything beyond hospital-based education classes given prenatally and immediately postpartum. Perhaps at six weeks postpartum outreach programs with home visits might help to support and counsel parents through difficult family developmental periods. Nursing research (Kutzner, 1984; Mercer, Hackley & Bostrom 1983; Weingarten, 1985) has demonstrated how mothers need support and counseling during the first three years of their child's development. Mothers and their children tend to be ignored unless alarming pathologies such as child abuse are evident. To date, there are little data to explain parental and/or sibling responses as well as their adaptation/coping strategies during the prenatal, intrapartal, and postpartal periods.

IMPLICATIONS FOR NURSING RESEARCH AND PRACTICE

Societal changes have influenced parenting and infant–child responses in the last 30 years. Mothers and fathers may or may not be involved in a marital or significant love relationship with each other, and children may or may not be integrated in their "birth" families or "blended" families. Traditional family patterns in childrearing are difficult to assess with so many varieties of familial groupings. Therefore, in modern society, questions and answers concerning the effects on children of significant developmental events such as the birth of a sibling are critical. Kagan (1980) has departed from traditional assumptions that parents should and must perform in certain ways to achieve a "successful" child. He suggests that "children do not require any specific actions from adults in order to develop optimally" (p. 129), and further states that there is no evidence to show that children are adversely affected by quantities of loving or discipline in order to become functional and happy adults. Kagan suggests that American children (1) need to believe that they are valued by their parents and a few special people from the community and extended family and (2) should develop autonomy, that is, the belief that they are able to and desire to make decisions regarding their conduct and their future, independent of coercive pressures from parents, teachers, and friends. Several concepts are therefore necessary to provide some uniformity for children with respect to their evaluation of parental acts of acceptance and rejection. Kagan suggests attention be given to the "attitude on the part of the parent, the quality and frequency of acts of parental care and stimulation, and the child's assessment of his values in the eyes of others" (p. 434).

What are the implications of these concepts for the parent with an older child, expecting another child? How does the parent portray these values to their older child and still experience the psychological and physical developmental changes during pregnancy? More important, is it possible for the health care provider to facilitate and support parents in achieving their goals?

Nursing research (Cronenwett & Wilson, 1979; Kutzner, 1984; Lederman et al., 1979; Mercer, 1980; Weingarten, 1985) has provided descriptive information regarding the relationship of nurses and families. The nurse assesses the parents and child(ren) initially within physical, psychological, social, and other criteria to ascertain baseline data. The nurse, utilizing a care-giving framework, interacts with the family to set goals and objectives of care.

Outside of standard prenatal, intrapartal, and postpartal criteria, the nurse can assess the child's reactions to the new sibling and engage in play and discussion actively, whether in a clinic, private office, or the family's home. At the same time, the nurse can observe the parents and child in a variety of situations and environments. With careful analyses of the parents' and child's interactions—perhaps enlisting criticisms from colleagues such as other nurses, physicians, and psychologists—the nurse and family can develop a strategy to support and prepare the child for the mother's pregnancy, labor, and delivery, and for the introduction of a new sibling. However, careful assessment of the child's general reactions to change and stress should be taken into consideration as well.

Dunn, Kendrick, and MacNamee (1981) examined the effects of the birth on the older sibling and found that most behavior problems disappeared by the time the baby was eight months old. They also found no association between the incidence of problems and the development of a poor relationship between siblings. Other studies that looked at children over a period of time found that fearful, worrying behavior in three- and four-year-olds that persisted over several years was associated with difficult behavior in eight-year-olds. An increase in anxious behavior after the sibling's birth was thought to be cause for concern. Dunn (1985) notes that children who have withdrawn after a sibling's birth may develop sibling relationships that are likely to be hostile and conflicted.

Dunn and Kendrick (1982a, 1982b) and Dunn et al. (1981) found that extreme forms of reaction were not associated clearly with ages of the firstborns at the birth, by sex of the child, or by whether or not the child was separated from the mother when she went to the hospital for the birth. They also noted that children younger than five years of age were more likely to become upset by the sibling's birth. The child's personality, however, is a more important factor than the age of the child, for children younger than five years, when determining reactions to the new sibling. That is, children who had patterns of labile emotions, difficult management, or inability to deal with change experienced the most difficulties with the birth of a sibling.

Dunn (1985) noted that the parent–child relationship was an important factor in the older child's reactions experienced in response to the sibling's birth. If a stable parent–child relationship were present, with close and supportive interactions, there was less reaction after the birth. Also, if mothers were extremely tired or withdrawn following the new baby's birth, the firstborn child was more likely to become withdrawn, probably in response to the mother's state.

While nurses can support and facilitate the child's adaptation and coping strategies during the pregnancy and birth of a new sibling, studies have not provided evidence that this preparation will decrease or avoid negative reactions by the older child. Mothers and fathers can be encouraged to prepare their children for the birth of a new sibling through individual family conferences or through parenting programs in the community or health facility. Dunn (1985) pointed out that, "however well prepared the child is, however clearly he seems to understand what the sibling's birth will entail, he may be overwhelmed by his emotional reaction to the event" (p. 115).

Again, the studies available in the literature do not provide information regarding sibling visitation in the immediate postpartum period. No association has been found between the child's first reactions to the sibling's birth immediately postpartum and subsequent behavior at home. Perhaps the nurse's best intervention involves preparing the mother and father for possible reactions, both positive and negative. Parents will be able to negotiate with their older children more effectively if they have some perception of possible behaviors. For instance, if the child becomes upset when the mother is feeding or changing the baby, perhaps the older child can be included in the infant's care directly. Some mothers collect toys and such to have on hand if the child becomes upset during care-taking activities, in order to distract the child and also show support for the child's other needs, thus providing the older sibling with assurances that her or his needs and desires are important to the parent.

Dunn and Kendrick's (1982a, 1982b) studies also suggest that mothers should avoid a sudden decrease in attention to their older children when the new baby is born. During the pregnancy, the parents can begin activities with their older child and encourage relationships with other children.

In summary, nurses can provide a supportive and educational atmosphere through their interactions with parents during pregnancy, labor and delivery, and the postpartum period. Although the research to date provides some explanations of the parents' and older children's responses to the new sibling's birth, individual family assessment remains critical to appropriate nursing interventions. An interdisciplinary approach is helpful in providing a forum for discussion and critique of patient/family approaches and strategies. Nursing research by Mercer (1986a, 1986b), Kutzner (1984), and Cronenwett (1983) describes how mothers appreciate and benefit from support from family, friends, and others during the first years of the child's development. Perhaps the nursing focus should include long-term follow-up in the first year, rather than the emphasis on the immediate postpartum period. Mothers may not be able to absorb and utilize information in large volumes in the first two to three days postpartum if they are physically and emotionally exhausted and withdrawn. Home visits by nurses during the six-week postpartum period and periodic telephone follow-up may provide a linkage with the caregiver that mothers and their families can utilize.

Although the emphasis on prenatal and postpartum education in acute-care centers is certainly positive, the mother's length of stay during the immediate postpartum period is decreasing rapidly due to early discharge programs developed by reimbursement agencies in order to decrease costs. It is even more critical that nurses provide continuity of care with telephone or home-visit follow-ups as well as coordination of community resources.

Finally, nurse researchers can address these issues with methodologies that begin to delineate nursing interventions and the effects on family interactions and development. Recent studies (e.g., Cronenwett, 1983) have demonstrated the effects of a postpartum support group during the first year after the birth of a child. Nurses need to study parents and their children over periods of time to assess short- and long-term effects of their interventions and the association of these interventions with health and cost outcomes. In addition, there are presently no data that provide cost information, either in regard to in-hospital nursing interventions or community follow-up. Nurses can more effectively provide safe and cost-effective care through further study of young families and their responses to developmental processes such as the birth of a second child.

REFERENCES

Bayley, N. (1969). *Bayley scales of infant development*. New York: Psychological Corporation.

Blake, J. (1981). The only child in America: Prejudice versus performance. *Population and Development Review, 1,* 43–54.

Bronfenbrenner, U. (1974). Developmental research, public policy, and the ecology of childhood. *Child Development, 45,* 1–5.

Bronfenbrenner, U. (1975, April). *Social change: The challenge to research and policy.*

Paper presented to the Society for Research in Child Development, Denver.

Bronfenbrenner, U. (1976). The experimental ecology of education. *Educational Researcher, 5,* 5–15.

Bronfenbrenner, U. (1977, March). *A theoretical model for the experimental ecology of human development.* Paper presented to the Society for Research in Child Development, New Orleans.

Bronfenbrenner, U. (1979). *The ecology of human development.* Cambridge, MA: Harvard University Press.

Bryant, B. K. (1982). Sibling relationships in middle childhood. In M. E. Lamb & B. Sutton-Smith (Eds.), *Sibling relationships: Their nature and significance across the lifespan.* Hillsdale, NJ: Lawrence Erlbaum Associates.

Cicirelli, V. G. (1977). Children's school grades and sibling structure. *Psychological Reports, 41,* 1055–1058.

Cicirelli, V. G. (1982). Sibling influence throughout the lifespan. In M. E. Lamb & B. Sutton-Smith (Eds.), *Sibling relationships: Their nature and significance across the lifespan.* Hillsdale, NJ: Lawrence Erlbaum Associates.

Clarke-Stewart, K. A. (1978). And daddy makes three: The father's impact on the mother and the young child. *Child Development, 49,* 466–478.

Claudy, J. G., Farrell, W. S., & Dayton, C. W. (1979). *The consequences of being an only child: An analysis of project talent data.* (Final Report No. NO1-HD-82854). Rockville, MD: Center for Population Research, National Institutes of Health.

Corter, C., Abramovitch, R., & Pepler, D. (1983). The role of the mother in sibling interaction. *Child Development, 54,* 1599–1605.

Cronenwett, L. (1983). *Relationships among social network structure, perceived social support, and psychological outcomes of pregnancy.* Unpublished doctoral dissertation, University of Michigan, Ann Arbor.

Dunn, J. (1983). Sibling relationships in early childhood. *Child Development, 54* 787–811.

Dunn, J. (1985). *Sisters and brothers.* Cambridge, MA: Harvard University Press.

Dunn, J., & Kendrick, C. (1979). Interaction between young siblings in the context of family relationships. In M. Lewis & L. A. Rosenblum (Eds.), *The child and its family.* New York: Plenum Press.

Dunn, J., & Kendrick, C. (1980). The arrival of a sibling: Changes in patterns of interaction between mother and firstborn child. *Journal of Child Psychology and Psychiatry, 21,* 119–132.

Dunn, J., & Kendrick, C. (1982a). *Siblings: Love, envy, and understanding.* Cambridge, MA: Harvard University Press.

Dunn, J., & Kendrick, C. (1982b). The speech of two- and three-year-olds to infant siblings: "Baby talk" and the context of communication. *Journal of Child Language, 9,* 579–595.

Dunn, J., Kendrick, C., & MacNamee, R. (1981). The reaction of first-born children to the birth of a sibling: Mothers' reports. *Journal of Child Psychology and Psychiatry, 22,* 1–18.

Falbo, T. (1982). Only children in America. In M. E. Lamb & B. Sutton-Smith (Eds.), *Sibling relationships: Their nature and significance across the lifespan.* Hillsdale, NJ: Lawrence Erlbaum Associates.

Kagan, J. (1980). The psychological requirements for human development. In A. Skolnick & J. H. Skolnick (Eds.), *Family in transition.* Boston: Little, Brown.

Kendrick, C., & Dunn, J. (1980). Caring for a second child: Effects on the interaction between mother and first-born. *Developmental Psychology, 16,* 303–311.

Klaus, M., & Kennel, J. (1970). Mothers separated from their newborn infants. *Pediatric Clinics of North America, 17,* 1015–1020.

Klein, M., & Stern, L. (1971). Low birth weight and the battered child syndrome. *American Journal of Diseases of Children, 122,* 15–18.

Koch, H. L. (1954). The relation of "primary mental abilities" in five- and six-years-olds to sex of the child and characteristics of his sibling. *Child Development, 25,* 209–223.

Kutzner, S. K. (1984). *Adaptation of motherhood from postpartum to early childhood.* Ann Arbor, MI: University Microfilms International.

Lamb, M. E. (1976). Effects of stress and cohort on mother- and father-infant interaction. *Developmental Psychology, 12,* 425–443.

Lamb, M. E. (1977). Father-infant and mother-infant interaction in the first year of life. *Child Development. 48,* 167–181.

Lamb, M. E. (1978). The development of sibling relationships in infancy: A short-term longitudinal study. *Child Development, 49,* 1189–1196

Lamb, M. E. (1979). The effects of social context on dyadic social interaction. In M. E. Lamb, S. T. Suomi, & G. R. Stephenson (Eds.), *Social interaction analysis: Methodological issues.* Madison, WI: University of Wisconsin Press.

Lamb, M. E., Suomi, S. T., & Stephenson, G. R. (Eds.). (1979). *Social interaction analysis: Methodological issues.* Madison, WI: University of Wisconsin Press.

Lederman, R. P., Lederman, E., Work, B. A., & McCann, D. (1979). The relationship of psychological factors in pregnancy to progress in labor. *Nursing Research, 132,* 94–97.

Lewis, M., & Rosenblum, L. (Eds.). (1979). *The child and its family: The genesis of behavior* (Vol. 2). New York: Plenum Press.

Mercer, R. T. (1980). Teenage motherhood: The first year; Part 1. Teenage motherhood: The teenage mother's views and responses; Part 2. How their infants fared. *JOGN, 9,* 16–27.

Mercer, R. T. (1981). A theoretical framework for studying factors that impact on the maternal role. *Nursing Research, 30,* 73–77.

Mercer, R. T. (1986a). The process of maternal role attainment over the first year. *Nursing Research, 35,* 10–14.

Mercer, R. T. (1986b). The relationship of developmental variables to maternal behavior. *Research in Nursing and Health, 9,* 275–285.

Mercer, R. T., Hackley, K. C., & Bostrom, L. (1983). Relationship of psychosocial and perinatal variables to perception childbirth. *Nursing Research, 32,* 202–207.

Nadelman, L., & Begun, A. (1982). The effect of the newborn on the older sibling: Mothers' questionnaires. In M. E. Lamb & B. Sutton-Smith (Eds.), *Sibling relationships: Their nature and significance across the lifespan.* Hillsdale, NJ: Lawrence Erlbaum Associates.

Parke, R. D., Power, T. G., & Gottman, J. (1979). Conceptualizing and quantifying influence patterns in the family triad. In M. E. Lamb, S. J. Suomi, & G. R. Stephenson (Eds.), *Social interaction analysis.* Madison, WI: University of Wisconsin Press.

Rubin, R. (1985). *Maternal identity and the maternal experience.* New York: Springer Publishing Co.

Sameroff, A. J. (1975). Early influences on development: Fact or fancy? *Merrill Palmer Quarterly, 21,* 267–294.

Sameroff, A. J., & Chandler, M. J. (1975). Reproductive risk and the continuum of caretaking casualty. In F. D. Horowitz, M. Hetherington, S. Scarr-Salapatek, & G. Siegel (Eds.), *Review of child development research* (Vol. 4). Chicago: University of Chicago Press.

Schachter, F. F. (1982). Sibling deidentification and split-parent identification: A family tetrad. In M. E. Lamb & B. Sutton-Smith (Eds.), *Sibling relationships: Their nature and significance across the lifespan.* Hillsdale, NJ: Lawrence Erlbaum Associates.

Sherwen, L. (1980). *An investigation into the effects of locus of control and psychoprophylactic method training on body cathexis and fantasy production in the primiparous woman.* Unpublished doctoral dissertation, New York University, New York, NY.

Wagner, M. E., Schubert, H. J. P., & Schubert, D. S. P. (1975). Sibship-constellation effects on psycho-social development, creativity, and health. *Advances in Child Development and Behavior, 14,* 57–148.

Weingarten, C. T. (1985). *Study of mothers of premature infants and mothers of full term infants: Their perceptions of their infants and the quality of their relationship with their husbands.* Unpublished doctoral dissertation, New York University, New York, NY.

Zajonc, R. B., & Markus, G. B. (1975). Birth order and intellectual development. *Psychological Review, 82,* 74–88.

Zigler, E., Lamb, M. E., & Child, I. L. (1982). *Socialization and personality development.* New York: Oxford University Press.

Chapter 10

Alternatives in Childbearing: Choices and Challenges

Carol Toussie-Weingarten and Jeanne Toussie Jacobwitz

Childbearing today in the United States has extended beyond the physiological process of reproduction into a multimillion-dollar industry aimed at the expanding family. As a result of professional and lay efforts, childbearing has come to be viewed as a critical period in the psychological evolution of the family. As the setting for most childbirths has shifted away from the home, the health care industry has taken on a larger role. Currently, factors such as professional and moral commitment toward family-centered childbirth and lively competition for obstetric patients among agencies have contributed toward the establishment of a variety of prenatal and delivery services. Today, the pregnant family is confronted with many choices and challenges within the health care system. By plan or by chance, each of these can affect the psychodynamics of the family.

This chapter will discuss the impact of the health care system on the psychological experience of the childbearing family. After consideration of some historical trends in childbearing, interventions and programs having impact on the psychological experience of pregnancy will be presented. Delivery alternatives available to pregnant families will then be noted in light of their advantages and limitations.

TRENDS IN CHILDBEARING:
THE EVOLUTION OF DELIVERY ALTERNATIVES

To appreciate the variety of childbirth alternatives today, it is important to consider the historical and social trends in childbirth that have evolved over the past century. No one individual or social factor quickly changed childbearing beliefs and practices; indeed, current practice reflects a complex and dynamic process. Today's alternatives in childbirth are the result of years of professional and lay groups' working together and against each other. No delivery alternative is universally accepted for the healthy pregnant family; however, the heterogeneous nature of the American population necessitates open availability of safe choices in childbearing. While the factors discussed in this section contributed to the evolution of parental choices in delivery they are not all inclusive. Readers with further interest are referred to obstetrical history sources for more in-depth discussion.

Prior to the twentieth century, almost all births in the United States took place outside of the hospital. Women were expected to deliver in a home setting where they would be attended by a woman experienced in childbirth, a midwife, or by a local physician. Limited transportation systems, limited availability of hospitals, and the state of hospital technology did not make hospital birth a ready option for most families. At this time, hospitals were generally considered the domain of the sick and infirm, not the place for women experiencing a normal life event. This trend continued into the beginning of the twentieth century.

Sociological and technological changes in the early twentieth century were accompanied by changes in patterns of obstetrical care and selection of place of birth. One major change was in the delivery attendant. For example, it was estimated that midwives delivered 38% of all babies in New York City in 1913 (Yankauer, 1983); however, there was subsequently a dramatic decrease in midwife-attended births. By 1935, the practice of midwifery was concentrated mostly among the poor and black populations in the rural South (Yankauer, 1983). Several factors may have contributed to this. The United States lacked educational programs for the training of skilled midwives[1]; at a time when women did not regularly enter the professions, there was a lack of women aspiring to be midwives. Unlike continental European countries where midwifery was considered an important subject requiring specialized education, the United States came to have no well-trained group of accoucheurs skilled in home births (Devitt, 1977). Through the early part of the twentieth century, immigrant women who came from societies where midwives normally attended home births continued this practice. With the advent of "modernization" and a desire to be upwardly mobile, many began to look toward the physician and the hospital as signs of prestige and of becoming American. At a time of complex medical advances, midwifery came to be opposed and physicians began to resent midwifery as an intrusion on the field of medical practice (Donahue, 1985; Gordon, 1982).

Midwifery was not completely eradicated, however. For example, the nurse midwife program begun in the early 1930s at the Maternity Center Association in New York City was physician sponsored. Among the formal and informal goals of the program were training midwives who would care for the poor and attempting to curtail the practice of lay midwifery. With the development of educational programs for nurse midwives, two groups of nonphysician birth attendants emerged in the United States; the nurse midwife and the lay midwife.

As defined by the Association for Certified Nurse Midwives (ACNM), a Certified Nurse Midwife (CNM) is

> an individual educated in the two disciplines of nursing and midwifery, who possesses evidence of certification according to the requirements of the American College of Nurse Midwives. . . . Nurse midwifery practice is the independent management of care of essentially normal newborns and women, antepartally, intrapartally, and/or gynecologically, occurring within a health care system which provides for medical consultation, collaborative management or referral. [Varney, 1980, p. 3].

---

[1]The American midwives of the eighteenth, nineteenth, and early twentieth centuries were lay midwives. It was not until 1911 that Bellevue Hospital established a school of midwifery. Nurse midwives first practiced in the United States in 1925, when Mary Breckenridge established the Frontier Nursing Service in rural Kentucky. This service was staffed by British midwives or American midwives educated in England or Scotland. It was not until 1931 that the Maternity Center Association in New York City opened the first school for nurse midwives in the United States (Donahue, 1985; Moore, 1983).

The philosophy of nurse midwifery focuses on childbirth as a natural, normal process and on assisting families to a safe and satisfying birth experience. After specialized training in obstetrics, nurse midwives must successfully pass a national certifying examination. Currently, CNM's are licensed by the state in which they practice. For example, in New Jersey CNM's are licensed by the New Jersey State Board of Medical Examiners, the same board that licenses physicians. In New York State, CNM's are licensed under the State Education Department; in still other states, CNM's are licensed under the state boards of nursing. Any restrictions on where CNM's may practice and the scope of their practice are decided by the individual states in which CNM's practice. Thus, the existence of a professionally educated, licensed group of birth attendants whose overall philosophy focuses on childbirth as a manifestation of health, rather than disease, offers a choice in childbirth attendant to the childbearing family. It was not until the late 1960s and early 1970s that nurse midwifery came into demand, educational programs for nurse midwives began to expand and increase in number, and nurse midwives became more widely available.

Lay midwives, on the other hand, are individuals who attend women giving birth but who are not nurse midwives or physicians. Their educational background varies widely, and it is not possible to identify a lay midwife as someone who has met a certain set of requirements to qualify to be a childbirth attendant. Indeed, some lay midwives may have had extensive apprenticeships and formalized training and may be able to care for pregnant families with great expertise. Other lay midwives may have very limited education or preparation for childbirth duties. While a few states have licensing requirements for lay midwives, their practice remains largely beyond the scope of professional regulation.

Lay midwives and nurse midwives do share a philosophy based on childbirth as a healthy, natural, family-oriented process. Confusion about these two different groups frequently arises, however, because of these philosophical similarities, because of the common title of "midwife," and because lay midwifery predated nurse midwifery in the United States.

Selection of the place for delivery also underwent change during the first half of the twentieth century. Although national statistics regarding place of birth were not available before 1935, there was a rise in rate of hospital births from 39.6% in 1935 to 96% in 1960 (Devitt, 1977). During this time, there arose a belief that pregnancy and birth were pathological phenomena, that is, disease entities that needed to be terminated, if necessary, by newly developed interventions such as use of forceps. Some of these interventions were believed to be more of a threat to patient well-being if practiced in a home, rather than a hospital environment. This contributed to physicians' support of hospital deliveries (Devitt, 1977). By 1930, obstetrics had emerged as a separate and important specialty of medical practice (Varney, 1980). The politics underlying this movement to establish obstetrics as a specialty further emphasized the presumably pathological nature of birth. In addition, obstetrical analgesia and anesthesia had come into use. Women were being told not only that they would be safer if they delivered in a hospital but also that they could experience a much less painful delivery there.

A reduction in the number of physicians during the first half of the twentieth century contributed to a heavier workload for existing physicians. During a period when the national birth rate was increasing and physicians were also being drafted into military service, concentrating obstetrical cases in hospitals allowed for more efficient use of a physician's limited time (Devitt, 1977). Then, in 1946, the Hill-Burton Act allocated funds for building hospitals in rural areas; thus, women who once had no choice other than home delivery could come into the hospital for their obstetrical care.

While changes were occurring in the type of birth attendants and place of delivery, changes in hospital procedures were also taking place. During the early twentieth century, strict isolation practices evolved from the high rate of morbidity and mortality of hospitalized children with communicable diseases. At the time it was thought that visitors brought the diseases, so visiting was minimized. To protect patients from the alleged illnesses of visitors, the practice of separating a hospitalized child from his or her parents came into being. This practice extended to the well-baby units, where infants were gathered into central nurseries and visiting by family members was greatly curtailed (Klaus & Kennell, 1982). Restrictions on contact between newborns and family members tended to persist, although evidence does not support the idea that extended contact between parents and their hospitalized newborns increases infections (Barnett, Leiderman, Grobstein, & Klaus, 1970; Urrutia, Sosa, Kennell, & Klaus, 1980).

By the middle of the twentieth century, just as at the start, there were few birthing alternatives available to the pregnant family; however, the psychodynamics of childbearing had moved nearly to the opposite pole. Power, choice, and decision making had become the domain of obstetrical health care providers and not recipients. By 1948 a woman could expect to have her pregnancy directed for her by her physician. If medications were needed, her pharmacist might not routinely identify them for her. At the time of labor, a woman would be brought to a hospital where she could expect to have her labor and delivery also directed for her. Analgesics and general anesthetics, along with interventions such as forceps, were widely used, even for routine deliveries, and their risks and benefits were not frequently discussed. A woman could expect to receive drugs with amnesic properties, not only for their sedative effects, but for their ability to prevent her recall of the painful events of labor. Images of the helpless, nervous father pacing a waiting room became a reality that provided subject matter for many a comic. Newborns were promptly removed to nurseries where they were cared for by masked attendants. Hospital personnel assumed all responsibility for infant care, and babies were permitted to be with their mothers only for feeding. The emphasis on health care technology and the establishment of hospital rules based on the potential pathology of childbirth made these practices so typical that when Grantly Dick-Read published *Childbirth without Fear* in 1944, he was thought radical.

Opposition to the mechanization of childbirth began in the 1950s; however, it did not gain momentum in the United States until the late 1960s, when the obstetrics pendulum began to swing in the direction of personalization in childbirth. Some of the greatest influences came from the women's movement. As women's groups banded together to pursue women's rights, importance came to be placed on women's understanding of and taking control over their own bodies. Criticism of standard hospital deliveries focused on factors such as lack of control over one's own body, lack of participation in decision making, rigidity of hospital rules, inability of women in the hospital to be surrounded by familiar support people during labor and delivery, and the emphasis on childbirth as a pathological experience.

By the 1970s, feminist groups were gaining strength and support. The issues of power and resistance to being controlled were presented to people in all parts of society through extensive media coverage;

childbirth was a recurrent theme. Feminists strongly argued that pregnancy for most women was a normal event and not a disease. Controversy began to focus upon preparation for childbirth, where to deliver, who the delivery attendant should be, and what choices women should have in childbirth. At the same time, back-to-nature and self-help groups began to focus on the natural aspects of childbirth and to press for childbirth settings and experiences that would promote these.

Prepared Childbirth

The prepared childbirth movement emerged from the belief that a woman's preparation for and active participation in labor and delivery was of psychological and physiological importance. As of the 1920s, a variety of behavioral methods to decrease perception of pain in childbirth had appeared. It was not until the late 1940s, however, during the post–World War II period of limited technological resources in the Soviet Union, that these were put into practice there. A lack of analgesics and anesthetics for women during parturition of necessity fostered greater reliance on more "natural" methods of dealing with pain in childbirth. These methods found greater use and acceptance in Europe and the Soviet Union than in the highly technologically oriented practices of American obstetrics.

Grantly Dick-Read, an English physician, had a major impact on the evolution of current choices in childbirth preparation that are available to American families. Dick-Read realized his belief in the emotional beauty of childbirth by developing a process of education and exercise that women could use to reduce their fears and, thus, muscular tension in childbirth. Through relaxation, the fear-tension-pain spiral could be prevented or inhibited (Dick-Read, 1944).

The psychoprophylactic method, based on principles first developed in the Soviet Union, was popularized by Ferdinand Lamaze, a French physician, and introduced into the United States in the 1950s. The main focus of techniques used in this method was the prevention of pain in childbirth through the use of the mind. This evolved from stimulus-response theory and suggested that women could learn to control their breathing and could be taught to relax in automatic response to the pain of contractions. Thus their perception of the pain would be altered.

The Kitzinger method, developed during the 1950s, used a psychosexual approach to pregnancy and childbirth (Bean, 1974). Developing her technique from a background in sociology and experience with different cultures, Kitzinger believed a woman needed to explore her feelings about her sexuality, her past experiences, and her relationship with her family. She encouraged active participation by the support person and also advocated marriage counseling as appropriate. Kitzinger's techniques differed from those Lamaze; for example, she did not believe in bearing down to push a baby out, but rather espoused gentle pushing techniques.

The Bradley method (Bradley, 1974), known as husband-coached childbirth, embodied a philosophy as well as a technique for childbearing. Bradley advocated the presence of the husband or lover at all times; he believed that a woman could best relax during contractions by reliving pleasant childhood memories that could then produce an automatic physical relaxation. Bradley emphasized that only the husband or lover could produce a mental relaxation in the laboring woman and therefore encouraged the male partner to remain at the woman's bedside at all times. Bradley also emphasized the need for "natural" childbirth, that is, birth without drugs in labor, good nutrition in pregnancy, and immediate contact between mother and child. Unlike the Lamaze program, which traditionally began during the last six weeks of pregnancy, the Bradley educational method began with weekly classes starting during the sixth month of pregnancy and continuing to term.

These examples represent only four of the childbirth-preparation methods that have been introduced. The various childbirth-preparation approaches differ from each other in the interpretation of why they work and in the basic activities that they teach, such as patterns of breathing. No one method, however, has been shown to work better than any other for all women (Bean, 1974). Today, a wide variety of childbirth-preparation programs exist, and many eclectic approaches incorporate aspects of different methods. Despite this variation, virtually all prepared-childbirth programs emphasize prenatal education and require both the laboring woman and a support person to be together. In addition, the woman must learn to relax her abdominal and vaginal muscles, breathe in a controlled manner, and use her muscles effectively in delivering the baby (Bean, 1974). A combination of physical and psychological techniques are used to assist a pregnant woman and her support person in dealing with labor in a personal way.

Regardless of the method advocated, the prepared-childbirth movement presents choices and alternatives to pregnant families. With the emphasis on factors such as little or no medication during normal delivery and a woman's active participation in delivery, the prepared-childbirth methods have departed from standard American hospital practices of the mid-twentieth century. They also have presented a challenge to a highly technologically oriented obstetrical system.

None of the methods in use today was widely welcomed in the United States; indeed, Dick-Read was considered a revolutionary (Yankauer, 1983). Women in the 1950s and early 1960s who elected to use "natural" childbirth frequently had difficulty in finding physicians willing to support them in the hospital. In addition, these women received opposition from staff and from other women. By questioning established practice, they were often seen as sacrificing the well-being of their infants for the politics of obstetrics.

By the mid-1970s, however, prepared childbirth had begun to gain widespread acceptance. The publicity received by childbirth-preparation techniques and the fact that studies could document positive psychological and physical outcomes of these methods for the pregnant couple also contributed to changing trends. Today, most American women have access to some type of childbirth-education program.

It is idealistic to think that hospitals and health care workers changed their focus for humanitarian reasons, away from major control of childbirth and toward encouraging patient responsibility and participation. As the public came to view childbirth as an opportunity for sharing between a couple, pregnant families began to seek out those settings and individuals who would assist them in safely orchestrating their own delivery. Economic concerns and sensitivity to consumer demands underlay policy and program changes in some institutions. If patients would keep coming, anything that was safe, feasible, and acceptable to the professional staff was fine.

A major limitation of any of the prepared-childbirth alternatives is the sense of failure that can be experienced by women who are unable to follow through with the programs they were taught. While some low-risk women are able to experience "easy" labors and deliveries, labor is a painful and difficult experience for others. Requesting and requiring pain medications is not a sign of failure. Indeed, childbirth educators need to emphasize that studying for exams in school and preparing for childbirth are not the same, despite attendance at scheduled classes. It is important for health professionals to address this topic specifically, as some women may not raise this concern prenatally.

The Cesarean Patient

Despite the availability of prepared-childbirth alternatives for low-risk women, by the late 1970s cesarean mothers were still being routinely treated as surgical patients. In most hospitals they were separated from their husbands for the delivery and denied the chance for active participation in a family-centered birth that mothers experiencing vaginal deliveries enjoyed. Through the organized efforts of cesarean mothers and concerned health care professionals and the establishment of organizations to represent the special emotional needs of the cesarean couple, childbirth-preparation programs for cesarean couples have been instituted. In addition, delivery options such as father's presence in the delivery room, use of epidural or spinal anesthesia to enable the woman to be awake for the delivery, and opportunities for early delivery- and recovery-room contact between parents and their newborn have been established.

Cesarean couples, however, still have only one choice of setting for delivery: a hospital. There currently continues to be great variation among hospitals regarding factors such as presence of husband during and after the cesarean delivery. The pregnant family should not assume that hospitals with advertised family-centered birth practices automatically extend these to cesarean patients. Pregnant couples should be encouraged to elicit this information from their physicians and/or the hospital prepared-childbirth coordinator, prior to their cesarean delivery. In light of the high rate of unplanned cesarean births, all pregnant couples should discuss with their caregivers during pregnancy what their emotional experience would be like in the event of a cesarean. Bing (1978) cautions against too much enthusiam for and acceptance of pleasant, family-centered cesarean births. She argues that it is the progressive rise in cesareans that should be questioned, rather than the methods for making them more desirable to the public by adding an attractive wrapper.

The possibility of a vaginal delivery for women who have previously had a cesarean delivery has emerged as a delivery alternative for some women. Fear of uterine rupture due to inability of scar tissue in the uterus to withstand the forceful contractions of labor has led to the belief that, once a woman has had a cesarean, she will always need one. Although uterine rupture is a major and life-threatening complication, its low potential incidence has made vaginal delivery an option for women who do not have recurrence of the condition requiring a cesarean section in their previous delivery; who begin labor before their estimated date of confinement; and who enter the labor suite with the fetal head well engaged and the cervix soft, effaced, and dilated at least 3 cm (Bobak & Jensen, 1984). However, the possibility of vaginal delivery after a cesarean is a decision that needs to be made on an individual basis and through discussion between a pregnant woman and her health care provider.

The Role of the Nurse in Prepared Childbirth

Nurses' roles in prepared childbirth include acting as sources of information and referral and as childbirth educators. It is thus essential for nurses to be aware of existing local programs and delivery settings that will support the choices pregnant families have made. Childbirth educators need to discuss the unpredictable nature of childbearing and to avoid giving families the impression that inability to follow a set method means failure.

Nurses in a labor and delivery setting need to know the type of method a couple has studied and to assess their mastery of that method through observation of their interactions in labor. Nurses should not assume that attendance in classes means expert knowledge; thus they should be prepared to do much on-the-spot coaching in a nonjudgmental manner. The nurse also needs to know the advantages and limitations of each method and to work with each couple to develop their confidence and trust. Undoubtedly, there will be occasions when a couple's delivery plans do not turn out as expected and unanticipated interventions, such as internal fetal monitoring or fetal blood scalp sampling, may be necessary. Thus, an important nursing role is to help families minimize the fear-tension-pain cycle and to have an optimal delivery experience, whatever technology is required.

A special relationship can develop between a couple and the nurse who assists them during childbirth preparation and delivery. In home or birth-center settings, there routinely is continuity of contact between the pregnant family and their birth attendants. It is also appropriate for this to occur in hospital; in many places, nurses need to take the initiative and visit on the postpartum unit those patients whom they have coached in labor. Childbirth educators can provide continuity through a postpartum reunion class or by telephone contact. A caring, interested approach on the part of the staff may be one reason why pregnant couples select certain alternatives in delivery settings.

IMPACT OF THE MEDIA ON THE PSYCHODYNAMICS OF CHILDBEARING

The media have great influence on the psychodynamics of pregnancy and on childbearing choices. According to Kalisch and Kalisch (1982), television is the single most important source of information in the United States. Quoting *U.S News & World Report's* seventh annual survey of "Who Runs America," they noted that television ranked second only to the White House in influence. In an editorial on birth control methods, Klein (1984) noted that levels of use of pills and IUD's went "up and down like a roller coaster" in relation to media reports of their adverse effects.

While word of mouth and professional referrals are certainly means of reaching potential patients, many clients come for services they have heard about through the media. The huge amounts spent on all sorts of paid advertising, as well as free coverage resulting from being the focus of a program, attest to the success of the media in attracting consumer patronage for all types of goods and services. Childbirth alternatives, which have received increasing coverage in television, newspapers, magazines, and radio reports, are no exceptions. By bringing issues and emotional considerations into the consumers' homes, the media have an important effect on dissemination of information about childbearing alternatives. By their manner of presentation, the media can also promote acceptance or rejection of current practice. It thus becomes essential for health care professionals working with pregnant families to keep themselves aware of ways in which childbirth and childbirth alternatives are being presented. Another appropriate role is for nurses to become involved in the media through active response to and production of programs dealing with childbearing.

CHILDBIRTH ALTERNATIVES

There are currently several childbirth alternatives in existence. Theoretically, couples are able to decide whether birth will take place in a hospital, in a birth center, or at home. They are also able to select either a physician, certified nurse midwife (CNM), or lay midwife as birth attendant. However, an appropriate choice for one family may be unacceptable for another. Decisions about where and with whom to deliver involve the interaction of complex factors such as a woman's past experiences, perceived risk factors, socioeconomic considerations, attitudes of significant others, availability of choices in her geographic area, and the goals for her birth experience (Hurzeler, 1985). Unfortunately, access to care and alternatives in childbirth may also depend on a family's ability to pay for the desired services. In some states, insurance companies may choose not to reimburse patients for deliveries anywhere but in a hospital. In addition, the full range of delivery alternatives and birth attendants often is available only for the low-risk obstetrical patient.

The Hospital Birth Experience

In theory, hospitals offer prenatal, intrapartal, and postpartal care to women at all levels of obstetrical risk. For high-risk women and women who require cesarean delivery, this is the only recommended alternative, and a physician is the primary birth attendant. Physicians still do the greatest numbers of all hospital deliveries; indeed, there are many fewer CNM's than physicians who practice obstetrics. However, increasing numbers of CNM's are obtaining delivery privileges and becoming active participants in hospital obstetric departments. Thus, low-risk women may be able to select either a physician or a CNM in many hospital settings.

Hospitals vary greatly in terms of services offered and capabilities for treatment of families at various levels of risk. They range from facilities able to handle only healthy mothers and infants to second-level facilities managing certain types of high-risk mothers and infants to tertiary-care settings able to care for those at highest risk. Regionalization of health care has resulted in the frequent transporting of sick newborns to a central facility, thereby separating mother and infant. These factors may be considerations for those families who live in areas where such choices exist.

The alternatives for birthing experiences in a hospital include laboring in one room with subsequent transport to a separate delivery room, or laboring and delivering in the same room. This room might be a traditional labor room or a specially equipped birthing room. Except in cases where operative procedures or general anesthesia are needed, and in situations where the level of risk to mother or fetus is great, there are few advantages in the traditional transport of a laboring woman to a delivery room. This practice is not only difficult for staff but uncomfortable and ill timed for patients. Indeed, Maloney (1980) found that elimination of transfer to a delivery room was considered by new mothers to be a major strength of their birthing-room experience. One standard argument for transfer of a labor patient to a delivery room focuses on the small size of labor rooms in older facilities and lack of available labor rooms for women on busy obstetric services. Both of these situations meet organizational needs, yet are not of psychological benefit to the family.

Hospital-based birthing rooms allow mothers to labor, deliver, and recover in one room; thus, a homelike birth experience can be simulated within the hospital setting. As such, the birthing room represents a hospital's attempts to integrate the family's psychological needs with the institution's goals. A support person may remain with the laboring woman; in some places siblings, other family members, or friends may also be present. Since labor and delivery occur within the same room, transport to a separate delivery area is eliminated. Should a change in maternal or fetal condition necessitate obstetric interventions, such assistance is nearby and accessible. Following delivery, there is opportunity for early and extended contact between parents and newborn within the same setting. Birthing rooms can include

1. A birthing bed, specially designed to accommodate different positions, the bottom half of which can be removed to facilitate the birthing process
2. Minimal visibility of medical equipment
3. Homelike furnishings such as a rocking chair, wall paper, cradle, television, and soft lighting
4. Private bath

Surveys of women using birthing rooms have shown consumer satisfaction with this type of birthing alternative (Dobbs & Shy, 1981; Faxel, 1980; Kieffer, 1980; Maloney, 1980). Indeed, from a study of 109 women, Kieffer (1980) found that 33% reported they would have delivered at home were it not for the presence of a birthing room.

Implementation of a homelike, personal delivery experience in birthing rooms has also had impact on policies used throughout obstetric units. For example, the application of antimicrobial ophthalmic preparations now is delayed, to promote parent-infant bonding through eye-to-eye contact. There is increased staff willingness to alter harsh lighting in delivery rooms, and the use of different birthing positions in the delivery room is more widely accepted (Faxel, 1980). The presence of a birthing room builds into the organizational structure of an obstetrical unit a mechanism for family-centered obstetric care, regardless of the level of obstetrical capability. Birthing-room practices need not be in conflict with highly technological practice. Healthy mothers and infants are common goals for care of patients, regardless of risk status. A family-centered approach, which this birthing alternative encourages, does not mean denying advances in obstetrics; rather, it means encouraging the appropriate types of intervention for each patient.

The presence of a birthing room in a hospital does not mean that it will be utilized as a delivery alternative. Hospitals may advertise beautiful birthing rooms as a means to attract patients; however, lack of support from regular staff nurses and physicians can effectively block this alternative for pregnant couples. For example, the possibility of complications can be used to bar women from the birthing room (Rothman, 1983), even those women who do not appear to be high risk. The attitudes and philosophy of the staff involved are essential for an emotionally satisfying hospital birthing-room experience (Maloney, 1980).

Criteria for use of a birthing room vary with each facility. Some institutions have very strict criteria (Averitt, 1980) and allow only women at very low risk to use the birthing room. Other facilities are more flexible in their admission criteria and allow most women who will deliver vaginally to use the birthing room, regardless of their risk status. Pregnant couples planning to use this alternative for labor and delivery thus need to find out whether their hospital has a birthing room and whether they would be considered likely candidates for using it.

At its best, the birthing room offers couples the opportunity to experience an emotionally supportive, homelike birth and yet have the back-up services that a hospital is able to provide quickly. In addition, the existence of birthing rooms highlights a change in obstetrical focus toward greater consumer participation in childbirth. However, inability to qualify to use a birthing room or need for transfer due to unforeseen labor complications can foster feelings of failure and frustration for some women.

The following list summarizes the advantages of birth in a hospital setting:

1. Feelings of security; availability of emergency equipment and treatment for mother and/or infant
2. Potential use of a birthing room; ability to combine homelike advantages of a birthing-room experience with security of delivery in an acute-care setting
3. Availability of professional staff to assist with birth
4. Availability of latest technology and staff who theoretically are able to use it effectively
5. A more sanitary environment in situations where heat, running water, and environmental hygiene are problems
6. For women with one or more children at home, a chance to spend some quiet time alone with the new baby and to rest
7. Contact with other new mothers and guidance from professional staff
8. Insurance coverage of birth expenses
9. Availability of analgesia and anesthesia, if needed

The disadvantages of birth in a hospital setting include

1. Care that can be impersonal, routine, and provided by many individuals the woman has never met prior to delivery
2. Potentially rigid hospital rules and regulations and variable interpretation by staff
3. Restrictive visiting policies for family and friends
4. Increased risk of unnecessary interventions, due to the disease orientation of hospital personnel
5. Use of unnecessary medications
6. Hospital limitation of options such as ambulating in labor, eating lightly, choice of delivery positions, and so forth
7. Separation from other children at home, necessitating extended child care assistance from family or friends

Freestanding Birth Centers

Birth centers are facilities that offer homelike birthing experiences outside a hospital. They are usually licensed by the states in which they are located. Some emergency equipment is available on the premises, and transportation to a back-up hospital is accessible.

Birth centers are usually decorated in a homelike fashion and have ample space for a woman's significant others. Indeed, in many birth centers women may have whomever they choose attend their births. Prenatal care may also be provided in the same center, so that a family becomes familiarized with the place where they will have their baby. The birth center may be owned by a physician, by CNM's, by lay groups, or any combination of these. Licensed facilities have physician consultation available as needed (DeJong, Kirkwood, & Carr, 1981).

Birth centers have grown in popularity, largely as a reaction to consumer perceptions of hospital birth. Nationally, 1 to 2% of births outside hospitals occur in birth centers, although there are reports that as many as 11% of women might be interested in this option (Lubic, 1985). Personal feelings of alienation, lack of control or involvement in decision making, and frustration with rigid hospital policies are among reasons consumers have sought an alternate birth experience. These are similar to the reasons consumers select in-hospital birthing rooms. According to Lubic, those families who felt alienated from in-hospital standard care were most likely to engage in professionally unattended home birth. Establishment of a birth center alternative thus effects a compromise between institutional and home birth.

In 1975, the Maternity Center Association in New York City became the first freestanding birth center in the United States. It has remained the prototype for American birth centers (Bennetts & Lubic, 1982). By 1981, the Cooperative Birth Center Network was formed to provide information on a national level and to help facilitate the establishment of birth centers (Lubic, 1985). It is estimated that there are currently more than 150 birth centers located in 32 states (Lubic, 1985). While consumer demand has been a strong factor in the opening of birth centers, their appeal extends as well to CNM's, as settings in which they have the power to practice full-scope midwifery.

Only low-risk women—those with no history or foreseeable possibility of medical, obstetrical, or psychiatric complications—can be accepted for care in a birth center. No one can be guaranteed that the birth will actually take place there, as a woman may be "risked out" prenatally or transferred intrapartally. It is therefore possible for families to experience a sense of failure and frustration as a result of not being able to actualize their birth plan. While it is not possible to identify rates of transfer accurately for all birth centers, rates of transfer as high 15% (Bennetts & Lubic, 1982) to 20% (Zabrek, Simon, & Benrubi, 1983) have been reported.

Delivery at a birth center requires active participation and assumption of responsibility on the part of the pregnant family. In a study done of 11 birth centers, Bennetts and Lubic (1982) documented a profile of birth center clients. The women tended to be in their mid-twenties (mean age 25), urban residents (64%), white (63%), married (88%), and motivated toward learning about childbirth (95% had taken prepared childbirth courses; 82% had attended at least nine prenatal visits). Cohen (1982) compared 30 women who selected a tertiary-care university obstetrical service with 30 women who chose an out-of-hospital alternative birth center staffed by nurse midwives. Women using the birth center tended to be more adaptable in preparation for their babies, perceived their partners as more supportive and involved in the birth, and intended to focus on autonomy and independence in their childrearing, compared to the group choosing the hospital. These women differ markedly from the poor, rural clientele served by midwives in the earlier part of the twentieth century (Yankauer, 1983).

The advantages of having a baby in a birth center include

1. Continuity of prenatal, intrapartal, and postpartal care
2. Comfortable, homelike setting
3. Opportunity for couple to participate actively in design of a personal birth plan
4. Wellness orientation; decreased chance of unnecessary obstetrical procedures or medications
5. Less expensive than delivery in hospital
6. Opportunity to become well educated about one's childbirth
7. Discharge within 24 hours and usually within 12 hours after delivery

The disadvantages of delivery in a birth center include

1. Possibility of transfer to another facility where birth center attendants may not be permitted to attend.
2. Appropriate only for healthy women at lowest risk; possibility of being "risked out" at any time during pregnancy or labor.
3. Limited accessibility; some patients may have to travel long distances for care or may not have this as a birth alternative.

4. Possibility of being transferred by ambulance during painful periods in labor.
5. Possibility of needing emergency interventions (e.g., cesarean delivery) not quickly available in a birth center; possibility that the delay during transfer may threaten healthy delivery outcome.
6. Cost may be higher if insurance does not cover deliveries planned for birth center.
7. Regional anesthetics not available; in some places, analgesics also not available.
8. Sense of failure experienced by some women unable to realize their birth plan, as a result of transfer to a higher-risk facility.
9. Need for active participation on the part of the pregnant woman in the prenatal and labor process would be a disadvantage for women unwilling or unable to assume this responsibility.

Home Birth

Although nearly all births occurred at home a century ago, today this is a childbirth alternative not used by most women. Because it is difficult to compile statistics on births at home, it is not possible to identify with accuracy the actual number of women selecting home delivery; however, we do know that there is great variation among those who have home births. The profile of people choosing home birth ranges from well-educated, older, multiparous women who have received complete prenatal and intrapartal care from a health professional, to poor, malnourished women with minimal or no prenatal care and no specialized birth attendants (DeClerq, 1984; U.S. Department of Health and Human Services, 1984). In 1984, the National Center for Health Statistics (U.S. Department of Health & Human Services, 1984) analyzed midwife and out-of-hospital deliveries from data obtained from birth certificates. The results identified three reasons why women select home birth:

1. The majority of women in the study delivered at home due to geographic reasons, that is, inability to get to a hospital.
2. The desire for a family-centered birth experience was often cited.
3. For some, the delivery came at home due to unexpected circumstances.

Arguments regarding the safety of home birth and the psychological benefits to the family have been cited by both advocates and opponents of home births. Again, it is difficult to make statistical comparisons due to the problems in obtaining data regarding out-of-hospital births. Birth certificates often do not specify whether the birth took place at home or in a birth center or whether it was a planned or unplanned home birth. While the birth attendant may be listed as a midwife, he or she may not be identified as a CNM or a lay midwife (Gregory, McDonough, Maciorowski, & Miller, 1984). Birthing centers, licensed by the state in which they operate, may be classified as hospitals; further confusing the issue (U.S. DHHS, 1984). Statistics are available from The Farm in Tennessee (Gaskin, 1977,); from home birth practices in Arizona (Sullivan & Becman, 1983); from Sweden, Denmark, Holland, and England (Adamson & Gare, 1980). These data indicate that home birth can be safe when appropriate back-up is available and trained birth attendants are used. As might be expected, women who receive prenatal care and obstetrical screening and who are attended at birth by trained professionals have better outcomes overall than women who have unattended home births (Burnett, 1980; DeClerq, 1984).

Mehl, Peterson, Whitt, and Hawes (1977) defend home birth as a safe alternative to hospital birth in certain selected, medically and obstetrically low-risk populations. They also cite lower cesarean rates, less need for forceps, and less use of anesthetics and oxytocics among these women than among those who have their entire labors and deliveries in hospitals. Those against home birth believe such comparisons are misleading, as couples who actively choose home birth tend to be highly motivated and self-selected (Adamson & Gare,

In an evaluation of home births in Santa Cruz County in California, Mehl, Petersen, and Shawn (1975) found that only 25% of home births were actually recorded, and these represented the home births with complications. Transfer rates of 10 to 33% have been cited among women having home births (Adamson & Gare, 1980; Mehl, Petersen, & Shawn, 1975). Opponents of home births believe this demonstrates the unpredictable nature of childbearing and that having a baby at home presents an unnecessary risk to mother and infant. They further attribute decreases in perinatal morbidity and mortality to the shift to hospital deliveries and use of technologies that have developed over the last 40 years (Adamson & Gare, 1980). Proponents of home birth argue that most complications can be predicted and that problems such as abruptio placenta and neonatal asphyxia are rare.

Clearly, the alternative of home birth is extremely controversial, and the nature of obstetrical complications and the lack of research studies focusing on the safety of home birth mean that this controversy will persist. The reality is, however, that consumers do continue to choose to give birth at home, so nurses need to be aware of the existence of this alternative.

In many states, lay midwives are primarily responsible for supervision of home births. Indeed, lay midwives do not generally have delivery privileges at hospitals or licensed birth centers. The home provides an environment in which they can practice without the credentials required by hospitals or licensed birth centers. Physicians and CNM's may be reluctant to participate in planned home births in areas where hospitals or licensed birth centers are readily available. In addition to questions as to the safety of home birth, physicians and CNM's may also be concerned about the possibility of malpractice suits brought as a result of unfavorable birth outcomes. Women committed to giving birth at home might therefore find their choices limited to a lay midwife or a theoretically unskilled birth attendant.

The advantages of home birth include

1. Potentially emotionally satisfying family experience
2. Ability for a woman to labor and deliver within her own familiar environment; no need to move to another facility for labor and delivery
3. Opportunity for couple to design their own birth plan
4. Wellness orientation; decreased chance of unnecessary obstetrical procedures or medications
5. Less expensive than delivery in hospital or birth center
6. Early, extended, and uninterrupted contact with newborn

The disadvantages of home birth include

1. Possibility of needing emergency interventions not available at home
2. Difficulty in finding qualified birth attendants
3. In cases of maternal, fetal, or neonatal emergency, transfer may

result in life-threatening delay, especially since access to appropriate transportation may be limited

4. Possibility that the expected birth attendant may be with another client, resulting in an unattended birth
5. Cost may be higher if insurance does not cover birth attendant's fees
6. Anesthesia and analgesia not available
7. Appropriate only for healthy women at lowest obstetrical risk

LITIGATION AND LIMITATIONS ON CHOICES IN CHILDBIRTH

A dramatic increase in malpractice suits brought against health care professionals in obstetrics has begun to emerge as a factor limiting choices in childbirth. A legal system that initially evolved to protect or compensate consumers for harmful professional acts of omission or commission has developed into a restrictive force that ultimately benefits neither consumers nor professionals as groups. Few would deny the need to compensate victims of malpractice or to remove the incompetent from practice; however, the current rash of lawsuits has had its impact on obstetrics and obstetrical nursing. The large claims awarded to plaintiffs, the reluctance of insurance companies to write insurance for obstetricians and nurse midwives, and the willingness of insurance companies to settle claims out of court simply because it may be less expensive than proving an obstetrician's, CNM's, or nurse's innocence through a court trial have contributed toward development of a high-risk approach toward childbirth. Another possible outcome may be more widespread use of technology, costly diagnostic testing, and surgical interventions such as cesarean deliveries, in order to prevent potential complications even in women who might otherwise have had normal labors and deliveries. Difficulty in obtaining malpractice insurance might not make it feasible for some freestanding birth centers to remain open, thereby limiting the availability of this birthing alternative. Ever-increasing costs of malpractice insurance premiums (to amounts approaching $100,000 annually) have been behind the decision of obstetricians in some areas to close their practices to new obstetric patients and to focus only on gynecology, a specialty judged to be at lower risk for huge malpractice settlements and therefore one in which malpractice insurance rates are much lower than obstetrics. CNM's, whose overall salaries are less than those of obstetricians, may also be priced out of the market by insurance premiums. The cost of premiums, passed along to consumers, can limit access to health care for some pregnant women who cannot afford the high fees. In addition, the publicity and professional frustration accompanying these situations may further deter potential health care professionals from specializing in care of the childbearing family. A long-term outcome of these circumstances may be a restricted supply of qualified childbirth attendants, with the resulting need for more women either to deliver at home or to travel long distances for care. These potential restrictions on childbearing alternatives raise major concerns for consumers and health care workers. Clearly, there is much need for collaborative efforts to find solutions that will allow obstetricians, CNM's, maternity nurses, and consumers to participate in a wide range of safe childbirth alternatives.

CONCLUSION

Today the importance of patient and family involvement in pregnancy and birth has become integrated with scientific technology. While debate persists as to the degree to which technology should be used for healthy, low-risk women, there is a trend toward making childbirth a family-centered experience, regardless of risk.

Preparation for childbirth has become so widely accepted in the United States that pregnant families are able to choose from a variety of methods and approaches offered by hospitals, birth centers, and independent childbirth educators. Some type of prenatal education is usually available to pregnant families, regardless of their socioeconomic status. Nurses have important roles as childbirth educators, as sources of referral for childbirth education, and as sources of support in enabling couples to use their childbirth-preparation methods in labor and delivery settings. Nurses working in childbirth settings thus need to be aware of various childbirth methods and approaches, the existence of childbirth-preparation programs in their community, and the ways in which these programs and alternatives are portrayed by the media.

Although several alternatives for delivery attendants and settings have been presented in this chapter, such a discussion is academic for many American couples. Many do not have the luxury of choosing an alternative childbirth attendant or setting and therefore, must use whoever or whatever is available. In addition, there are only about 2,000 CNM's practicing in the United States and less than 200 free-standing birth centers. While this represents an increase in alternatives that were available a decade ago, in no way can such a small number be accessible to most American families. Thus, physician-attended hospital and out-of-hospital births will continue to be the primary choices available to American women. Within the context of a hospital, the birthing room offers the physical setting most likely to provide a homelike birth experience.

The alternatives in childbearing that have emerged highlight the desire of consumers for emotionally supportive, family-centered childbirth experiences. The out-of-hospital and midwife-attended alternatives, as well as use of in-hospital birthing rooms, pertain to those women at low obstetrical risk. Every pregnant family, however, has the right to supportive, safe, and personalized care. A challenge to all nurses is to identify the psychological factors that have sparked the need for birthing alternatives and to strive to make childbearing experiences as psychologically supportive as possible for families, regardless of risk or setting.

REFERENCES

Adamson, G. D., & Gare, D. (1980). Home or hospital births? *Journal of the American Medical Association, 243,* 1732–1736.

Averitt, S. S. (1980). Adapting the birthing center concept to a traditional hospital setting. *Journal of Obstetric, Gynecologic and Neonatal Nursing, 9,* 103–108.

Barnett, C. R., Leiderman, P. H., Grobstein, R., & Klaus, M. H. (1970). Neonatal separation: The maternal side of interactional deprivation. *Pediatrics, 45,* 197–205.

Bean, C. (1974). *Methods of childbirth.* Garden City, NY: Doubleday.

Bennetts, A. B., & Lubic, R. W. (1982). The free-standing birth centre. *Lancet, 8268,* 378–380.

Bing, E. (1978). Correspondence. *Birth and the Family Journal, 5,* 105.

Bobak, I., & Jensen, M. D. (1984). *Essentials of maternity nursing.* St. Louis: C. V. Mosby.

Bradley, R. (1974). *Husband coached childbirth.* New York: Harper & Row.

Burnett, C. A. (1980). Home delivery and neonatal mortality in North Carolina. *Journal of The American Medical Association, 244,* 2741–2745.

Cohen, R. L. (1982). A comparative study of women choosing two different childbirth alternatives. *Birth, 9,* 13–19.

DeClerq, E. (1984). Out of hospital births, U.S., 1978: Birth weight and Apgar scores as measures of outcome. *Public Health Reports, 99*, 63–72.

DeJong, R. N., Kirkwood, K., & Carr, K. C. (1981). An out of hospital birth center using university referral. *Obstetrics and Gynecology, 58*, 703–706.

Devitt, N. (1977). The transition from home to hospital birth in the United States. *Birth and the Family Journal, 4*, 47–58.

Dick-Read, G. (1944). *Childbirth without fear*. New York: Harper.

Dobbs, K. B., & Shy, K. K. (1981). Alternative birth rooms and birth options. *Obstetrics & Gynecology, 58*, 626–631.

Donahue, M. P. (1985). *Nursing, the finest art: An illustrated history*. St. Louis: C. V. Mosby.

Faxel, A. M. (1980). The birthing room concept at Phoenix Memorial Hosital: Part I: Development and eighteen months' statistics. *Journal of Obstetric Gynecological Neonatal Nursing, 9*, 151–154.

Gaskin, I. M. (1977). *Spiritual midwifery*. Summertown: Book Publishing Company.

Gordon, I.T. (1982). The birth controllers: Limitations on out-of-hospital births. *Journal of Nurse-Midwifery, 27*, 34–39.

Gregory, M., McDonough, R., Maciorowski, L., & Miller, E. (1984). Out of hospital births: A survey of parents. *Journal of the Medical Society of New Jersey, 81*, 549–553.

Hurzeler, C. (1985). Finding a qualified home-birth attendant. *Genesis, 7*, 14–26.

Kalisch, B., & Kalisch, P. (1982). Nurses on prime-time television. *American Journal of Nursing, 82*, 264–270.

Kieffer, M. J. (1980). The birthing room concept at Phoenix Memorial Hospital: Part II: Consumer satisfaction during one year. *Journal of Obstetric, Gynecologic and Neonatal Nursing, 9*, 55–164.

Klaus, M., & Kennell, J. (1982). *Parent-infant bonding* (2nd ed.). St. Louis: C. V. Mosby.

Klein, L. (1984). Unintended pregnancy and the risks/safety of birth control methods. *Journal of Obstetric, Gynecologic and Neonatal Nursing, 13*, 287–289.

Lubic, R. (1985). Free standing birth centers: Where are we now? *Genesis, 7*, 11–13.

Maloney, J. (1980). The birthing room: Some insights into parents' experiences. In L. Sherwen & C. Toussie-Weingarten, *Analysis and application of nursing research: Parent-neonate studies, 1983*. Monterey, CA: Wadsworth Health Sciences.

Mehl, L., Peterson, G. H., & Shawn, S. (1975). Complications of home birth: An analysis of a series of 287 home births from Santa Cruz County, California. *Birth and the Family Journal, 2*, 123–135.

Mehl, L., Peterson, G. H., Whitt, M., & Hawes, W. (1977). Outcomes of elective home births: A series of 1146 cases. *Journal of Reproductive Medicine, 19*, 281–290.

Moore, M. L. (1983). *Realities in childbearing* (2nd ed.). Philadelphia: W. B. Saunders.

Rothman, B. K. (1983). Anatomy of a compromise: Nurse-midwifery and the rise of the birth center. *Journal of Nurse-Midwifery, 28*, 3–7.

Sullivan, D., & Becman, R. (1983). Four years experience with home birth by licensed (lay) midwives in Arizona. *American Journal of Public Health 73*, 641–645.

Urrutia, J. J., Sosa, R., Kennell, J. H., & Klaus, M. H. (1980). Prevalence of maternal and neonatal infections in a developing country: Possible low-cost preventive measures. *Perinatal Infections: Ciba Foundation Symposium 77.* Amsterdam: Excerpta Medica.

U.S. Department of Health and Human Services. (1984). *Midwife and out of hospital deliveries, United States.* Series 21, No. 40. Washington, DC: U.S. Public Health Service, National Center for Health Statistics.

Varney, H. (1980). *Nurse midwifery.* Boston: Blackwell Scientific Publications.

Yankauer, A. (1983). The valley of the shadow of birth. *American Journal of Public Health, 73,* 635–638.

Zabrek, E., Simon, P., & Benrubi, G. (1983). Nurse midwifery prototypes; clinical practice and education: The alternative birth center in Jacksonville, Florida—The first two years. *Journal of Nurse-Midwifery, 28,* 31–36.

Chapter 11

Trends in Research and Health Care Delivery to Pregnant Families

In the past 5 to 10 years, there has been dramatic change in delivery of health care, in both the public and private sector and to both pregnant women and newborn infants. The advent of state block grants for health care from the federal government and the use of diagnostic related groupings (DRG's) to reduce health care costs have produced the need to economize in delivery of care and to set priorities in expenditures for health and illness. In addition, the aging of the population has resulted in a burgeoning new area of health care in gerontology or geriatric practice which provides significant competition for federal and state health care dollars. For all of these reasons and more, care given to childbearing families has altered in focus (Flemming, 1985). How has this realignment affected childbearing families? This final chapter will briefly look at some current trends and statistics concerned with childbearing, in an effort to ascertain some objective answers to this question. In addition, it also will pinpoint some major issues in the area of maternity care and in maternity research conducted by nurses and others. Finally, the evolving role of the nurse in delivery of care to pregnant women and infants will be considered.

CARE OF CHILDBEARING FAMILIES
IN THE PUBLIC SECTOR

The debate over what is considered appropriate funding by the federal government concerning the health care delivery to mothers and children appears to focus on at least two major concerns. First, the infant mortality rate remains high in the United States, compared to other industrialized countries. The most recent statistics, published in 1985 (March of Dimes, 1985), ranked the United States seventeenth among countries, with an infant death rate of 11.2 per 1,000 live births. Our rate of decrease since 1972 was calculated at 39.5%. These statistics can be compared with Finland, the country with the lowest infant death rate. In 1982, Finland's rate was 6.5 deaths per 1,000 live births, with a decrease since 1972 of 42.5%. For a country with the resources of the United States, this infant mortality rate is seen as unacceptable (March of Dimes, 1985). Thus, there is concern at the federal level with reducing our infant mortality rate.

The second concern is our large federal budget deficit. Spending for health care in general seems to be seen as one area that requires reductions, and programs offering care to mothers and infants certainly are affected by this concern.

Funding Mechanisms and Funded Programs

There are two main ways that the federal government supports care of mothers and infants: indirect and direct support. Indirect sources of support include efforts to educate prospective parents, pregnant women, and health professionals through federally funded media, literature, or other educational programs.

Direct sources of support are the major programs that offer health care services to pregnant women and children. There are two main programs functioning as health care providers for women and children (usually limited to those individuals who cannot afford private care sources): (1) Medicaid and (2) Title V Maternal and Child Health Block Grants. Medicaid pays for health care services for over 10 million poor childbearing and childrearing families who have little or no health insurance. The Title V block grants provide states with funding to establish community health centers providing services to mothers and children who live in areas underserved by private providers, or who cannot afford private health care. It is approximated that 17 million pregnant women and children received health care services through the Title V Maternal and Child Health Block Grants (Collins & Natapoff, 1984).

In 1981, the Omnibus Budget Reconciliation Act established the block grants. This act redistributed federal monies, as direct grants, to the states, allowing states to determine their own funding priorities. By shifting money in "blocks" to states, it was theoretically possible to reduce spending through a reduction in administrative costs. Further, it was reasoned, the states could perceive their own health priorities better than the federal government. However, some of these reasonable thoughts were offset by a 25% reduction in total health funding levels (Collins & Natapoff, 1984). Programs for mothers and infants had to compete with other programs in each state for greatly reduced funds.

One additional source of federal support, separate from Medicaid and the federal block grants, is the Special Supplemental Food Program for Women, Infants, and Children (WIC). This program, enacted by Congress in 1972, provides prescription food packages and nutrition education to some 2 million pregnant women, infants, and children who are below a certain income level and who are found to be at nutritional risk.

In general, these programs funded by the federal government can be seen to direct care primarily at the high-risk mother and fetus. This might be seen as an attempt to improve our ranking among industrialized nations in terms of our infant mortality rate. This focus on the high-risk pregnancy becomes more evident when one considers that pregnant women at risk are defined both medically and sociologically. Medical risk factors include such conditions as kidney or heart disease, pregnancy-induced hypertension, diabetes, and so on. Sociological risk factors, however, include such factors as race (black or other minority), low socioeconomic status, age (teenagers), being a single parent, and so on. When one considers that often those risk factors seem to have an interactional effect, one can see that programs aimed at the poor are truly programs designed to improve outcomes of the high-risk pregnancy.

Changes in Federal Funding

Since the enactment of the block grants and budget cuts, various groups have attempted to monitor the effects of these funding changes on delivery of health care and other supports to mothers and children. A summary of their findings (Collins & Natapoff, 1984) includes the following:

1. Every state (10%) has reduced its Medicaid program for mothers and children by cutting back on services or making eligibility more difficult.

2. Forty-seven states (94%) report cutbacks in Title V Maternal and Child Health Block Grant programs during 1982 by reducing eligibility and/or health services.
3. Because of federal cuts affecting 239 community health centers, or 28% of all CHC's in the nation, 725,000 people, 64% of whom are children and women of childbearing age, have lost services at CHC's.

In an analysis of studies and papers designed to monitor effects of funding changes, Hussey and Scoloveno (1984) report that, in 1982, 19% of non-Title V categorical programs were cut. In 1983, an additional 28% of these programs were cut nationally. State-run Title V block grant services were cut 6% in 1982. However, in response to public outcry, these services were slated to be increased in the 1983 funding year.

WIC is also in danger from federal budget cuts. Studies have documented improvements in pregnancy outcome in women enrolled in WIC; however, this program currently is able to reach only one out of seven eligible individuals (Gartmaker, 1979). Proposed reductions in the WIC budget, believed by some to be as high as 33%, will greatly curtail the number of pregnant women and children eligible for these services. Such cuts have the potential to impact negatively on the nutritional status of pregnant women and in turn worsen the infant mortality rate.

Thus, the health care priorities of the federal government concerning pregnant women and neonates seem to coincide with changes in federal funding patterns. The focus would appear to be on the high-risk pregnancy and neonates (either due to medical or social factors), for these are the situations that produce high infant mortality statistics. Further, since monies are more limited, states and the federal government are beginning to channel scarce funds into programs that deal with the high-risk pregnant woman and neonate. Thus, programs deemed "unnecessary" or not having such an impact on high-risk pregnancies are loosing funding. Only the programs that can empirically document their effectiveness at reducing the infant mortality rate or improving pregnancy outcome will remain viable. Such a concern with documentation of programs will also affect federal funding of research.

CARE OF CHILDBEARING FAMILIES IN THE PRIVATE SECTOR

In response to federal priorities for the allocation of monies, the private sector has also appeared to direct its health care focus on similar areas. A major and growing concern of hospitals, physicians, and nurses who deal with childbearing is the high-risk pregnant woman and high-risk neonate.

Perinatology

In an effort to improve our national statistics concerning mortality and morbidity of neonates and infants, a major thrust of care has been aimed at the perinatal period, that is, the time surrounding the birth of the infant. The focus of such health care is on two types of patient: (1) the maternal-fetal unit (high-risk pregnant women and their unborn fetuses in utero) and (2) the sick neonate. This focus has spawned a multitude of new technical devices and instruments designed for the diagnosis and treatment of the high-risk fetus and neonate, advances in managing maternal conditions such as diabetes or toxemia, and several new specialties in both nursing and medicine. On many medical staffs, one now finds a perinatologist, neonatologist, or fetologist. Nurses are becoming certified in acute care of high-risk neonates and are trained in a variety of special perinatal inservice programs. Further, many colleges of nursing are evolving tracks within their graduate programs to offer nurses master's degrees in the specialty area of perinatal nursing.

Another consequence of the specialty of perinatology on care delivery during the childbearing period is the regionalization of high-risk care to mothers and infants. In each state, certain hospitals (designated "Level III" institutions) offer care to the most critically ill pregnant women and neonates. These individuals are transferred from local sites in the state to the designated hospital having a neonatal intensive care unit (NICU). Other hospitals having maternity services are designated "Level II" institutions; these have intermediate nurseries where sick infants and premature infants who are not critically ill may be cared for. Level I institutions are those hospitals having normal

rn nurseries. The safe transportation of critically ill mothers and
.... s has also become an issue in health care.

Care of the Neonate

Technological advancements aimed at caring for high-risk neonates
are allowing babies who would have inevitably succumbed five years
ago to survive and recover. Nurses, in collaboration with physicians,
are becoming highly skilled in a multitude of techniques and skills designed to stabilize acutely ill and very-low-birth-weight neonates. Prenatal diagnosis, consisting of fetal heart rate monitoring, ultrasound
scanning, fetal blood sampling, and biophysical profiling, alerts caretakers to potential problem areas before the infant is born. While nurses cover all phases of caring for sick infants, their major independent
role is working with the family of the high-risk neonate.

While nurses cover all phases of caring for sick infants, their major
independent role is working with the family of the high-risk neonate.
While technology may insure survival of a sick neonate, it cannot insure an intact family or an absence of emotional sequelae for the baby.
The nurse may be the primary support system and educator for the
family of the infant who has an extended stay in the NICU. It is up to
the nurse to insure that parents become acquainted with and attached
to their baby and eventually become confident in his other care.

Although technological advancements in care of high-risk neonates
seems to have accounted for a drop in rates of neonatal mortality and
morbidity, the drop in rates is slowing down. Some observers feel that
this is because the limit of improvements due to technology has been
reached. It is also known that many of the devices used to diagnose and
treat high-risk fetuses and infants are very expensive and become
dated quickly. Thus, another focus in care during the childbearing
period, and one perceived as possibly more important in the long run,
is the prevention of the birth of high-risk infants.

Prevention of High-Risk Births

There are several areas in health care delivery that have been
targeted as factors in the goal of preventing the high-risk birth. Premature births and low-birth-weight in infants are seen as the most important causes of infant mortality and morbidity. Thus, health care providers are directing much attention toward methods of identifying
those women at risk for these problems, and toward programs and
protocols designed to prevent occurrence of these births.

Health care delivery aimed at pregnant teenagers is also in response to the need to prevent high-risk births. Teenagers are at risk for many pregnancy complications and have a high incidence of sick infants. They also are often poor parents, and the psychosocial effects of teenage parenting produce sequelae for both mother and child. Programs are generally aimed at preventing adolescent pregnancy, ensuring a better pregnancy outcome, and improving the teenage mother's ability to parent her infant.

Many maternal conditions in the high-risk pregnancy, such as diabetes, can produce birth defects and other long-term sequelae for offspring. Low birth weight and prematurity are also associated with long-term effects on the child, both physical and psychological. In addition, many types of exposure during pregnancy—such as to environmental toxins, smoking, or alcohol—can produce birth defects. Education of pregnant women and excellent management of maternal conditions during pregnancy are health provider concerns in helping to reduce birth defects in neonates and the long-term effects of a high-risk birth. In addition, such nursing management techniques as infant stimulation in the NICU are aimed at reducing the impact of a high-risk birth on subsequent infant development.

Nutritional management of the pregnant woman is seen as a major way to help prevent low-birth-weight infants. Maternal nutrition is also more controllable than other factors of sociological risk; hence it is more accessible to professional intervention.

Finally, a focus of health care providers working in the area of childbearing is delivery of care to poor and minority families. The black population has a higher infant mortality rate than does the white poulation. High infant mortality is also associated with poverty. Many facets of the definition of high risk due to sociological factors are found in poor and minority populations. Thus, health care providers, if they truly are to impact on high-risk births—must devise appropriate care strategies for reaching poor and minority culture families.

The Low-Risk Birth

The private health care sector still has much concern for the low-risk birth situation, since this population generally "pays the bills." The previous chapter discussed current methods and issues in birthing. The intent here is to point out the seeming paradox in health care provider approaches to the low-risk pregnant woman and her family. On one hand, the woman and her mate are encouraged to be active participants in the birth, to use techniques to "stay in control" of the labor, and generally to experience a vaginal birth as a beautiful, natural event. On the other hand, parents are faced with obstetrical use of every available technology used in management of high-risk pregnancies. Some obstetricians advocate ultrasound scanning for every pregnant woman. Most hospital labor units now monitor fetal heart rate on every woman in labor, regardless of risk status. Such widespread monitoring has been linked to an increase in the cesarean delivery rate. Some individuals advocate the philosophical stance that cesarean delivery, due to its prevalence, should be considered as an "alternative birth method."

There are obviously advantages and disadvantages to both philosophical stances (natural versus technological) concerning birthing. The health professional and client might often stand on opposite sides in considering these two modes of birthing. Since there is no resolution to this issue at present, it will continue to be a focus of health care delivery for the low-risk pregnant client.

ETHICAL AND LEGAL ISSUES

Closely aligned to the last area of concern in health care delivery to childbearing families is a whole myriad of issues related to legal and ethical practices (Flemming, 1985). Again, it is not within the scope of this chapter to investigate these issues. The intent here is to alert the reader to the tremendous concerns that plague health care providers in the legal and ethical realms of delivering care to pregnant women and infants.

It is safe to say that most obstetricians, pediatricians, and specialists dealing with perinatal medicine practice "defensive medicine." Perceived mismanagement of labor and delivery can result in massive lawsuit awards. Hence, the physician is often quick to halt a labor that is not going according to the textbook, or one in which the fetal monitor picks up what could be interpreted as "fetal distress." The answer in this instance is to intervene with cesarean delivery; hence the greatly elevated cesarean birth rate.

Treatment of the sick neonate is also very risky, as attested to by the recent court awards to children for blindness due to retrolentalfibroplasia. In these cases, at the time these children were born, high oxygen concentration was the treatment of choice for premature infants with idiopathic respiratory distress syndrome (hyaline membrane disease). This treatment had the unfortunate side-effect of producing blindness in the infant. This practice, however, was based on the state of knowledge available at the time. If one can be said to be mismanaging care of an infant on the basis of knowledge yet undiscovered, then one is in great jeopardy.

While physicians are the prime targets of lawsuits, nurses who now participate in care regimens more and more as equal members of an interdisciplinary team will be more frequently included in such lawsuits. It is imperative that perinatal nurses become more sophisticated concerning legal aspects of the care they deliver to pregnant and laboring women and to sick neonates.

Ethical issues in health care delivery to childbearing families are also dramatic and in the forefront of public attention. Of course, the issue of abortion is still a tremendous controversy, especially with the position taken against it by the Reagan administration.

Other major ethical concerns surround the idea of informed consent for procedures on newborns and infants. Obviously, newborns cannot speak for themselves. Parents may be under stress and highly unreliable as informed consenters for procedures during the perinatal period.

A third major ethical concern of caregivers is the withholding of extensive "heroic" care, or even basic care, from presumably dying newborns. Should the nurse follow the planned regimen of withholding food from an ancephalic infant? This and many other similar issues will constantly face nurses and other health care providers working in the area of perinatal care, especially as technology advances and allows us to maintain some form of life in just about everyone.

NURSING RESEARCH FOCUS DURING CHILDBEARING

Nurses, like other researchers, vie for funding from federal and private sources to support their projects. Thus, in an effort to develop potentially "fundable" projects, research often closely parallels national priorities in care. Nursing research into the childbearing period has taken a swing to the perinatal or "acute care" arena. Especially favored are projects that investigate care protocols that will impact on pregnancy outcome and the recovery of sick neonates, or will save money in care of the high-risk mother or infant.

Research into High-Risk Conditions and Effectiveness of Care Practices

This area of research attempts to help the practitioner understand a particular high-risk situation or condition in the mother or infant and/ or looks at protocols for care that might impact on a partcular high-risk situation. The following is a necessarily incomplete list suggesting some research priorities and trends:

1. Research into care protocols or prenatal practices that improve pregnancy outcome includes studies on nutrition during pregnancy, causes/prevention of low birth weight in infants, and causes/prevention of premature labor.
2. Research into teenage pregnancy/abortion includes psychological "causes" and sequelae, improving pregnancy outcome, pregnancy prevention, improving parenting abilities, and effects on child growth and development.
3. Studies on the care of the high-risk neonate and the sequelae of being in a high-risk situation include use of infant stimulation and analysis of the long-term affects of the NICU environment.
4. Research into the care of the high-risk family includes examining parental perception/attachment to the sick neonate; family stressors in the high-risk situation (prenatal, labor/delivery, neonate, pueperium); the effects of transporting mother and/or infant; and long-term family sequelae.
5. Studies of early discharge/home care of the high-risk neonate examine care of the sick neonate at home, especially nursing management, and the economic/psychological benefits of early discharge.

Research into Practitioners of Maternal-Child Health Nursing

It is not only nurses who practice in the area of high-risk perinatal nursing who are of research interest; indeed, all practitioners of maternity nursing are coming under the researcher's scrutiny. Spurred by apparent gaps in graduate nurses' ability to deliver care to high-risk mothers and infants, the March of Dimes Birth Defects Foundation, American Nurses' Association (ANA), Nurses Association of the American College of Obstetricians and Gynecologists (NAACOG), and American Association of Colleges of Nursing (AACN) are sponsoring a federally funded project to develop maternal-infant nursing competencies that should be included in undergraduate curricula in baccalaureate nursing programs (Raff, 1984). Part of this project will study what currently exists in colleges of nursing, through a descriptive survey, in an effort to determine what is missing. Thus, education of the generalist and its efficacy in producing nurses who function in the specialty of maternal-child health nursing is being directly scrutinized. This area is also a federal priority.

Some other areas of research into the practitioners of maternal-child health nursing are nurses' reaction to and management of stress in the NICU, the nurse's role in working with high-risk families and parents in the NICU, and the nurse's role on the interdisciplinary team.

Research into Theories Concerning the Childbearing Family

Although funding might not be as abundant for nursing research in this area, many investigators are still interested in building and strengthening nursing theories that deal with the childbearing family and its members. It is felt by many that only through strengthening theory will adequate practice in nursing emerge. Some researchable areas in this category are

1. Pregnancy effect on family dynamics
2. Family or individual psychosocial factors related to high- or low-risk status
3. Parent-child interactions in normal and high-risk situations, including attachment versus separation-individuation, the effects of parental employment, and so on
4. Fathers and fathering during childbearing and childrearing, including role development, psychological state during pregnancy, and paternal nurturing activities

The foregoing is by no means a complete listing concerning current research efforts or areas of future research; however, it is hoped that it will stimulate the reader to evolve new concerns for nursing research in the area of the childbearing family.

THE NURSE'S ROLE IN PRACTICE AND RESEARCH

Previous chapters have discussed the nursing role and nursing interventions with the childbearing family. To summarize, it is seen that the

maternal-child heath (MCH) nurse has two basic types of roles—
either independent and interdependent. The same division holds true
for research as well.

A previous chapter discussed the nurse's independent role during
the childbearing period. The certified nurse midwife (CNM) and the
clinical nurse specialist (CNS) have both evolved independent roles in
delivery of care to pregnant women, neonates, and families. The CNM
manages low-risk pregnancies and deliveries. The CNS can manage
and coordinate care given to pregnant families, with special emphasis
on the psychosocial dimension.

In the realm of research, the majority of nursing research into
maternal-child health requires the independent effort of one or more
nurses. With the advent of the interdisciplinary perinatal health care
team, however, new forms of nursing research are emerging and will
be discussed.

The newest role for the MCH nurse, in both practice and research, is
that of an equal (or nearly equal) member of an interdisciplinary team.
In the past, nurses worked under the direction of physicians in the
realm of acute care. The discipline of perinatology, however, is perceived as so complex that many professionals are believed to be
necessary to manage the high-risk pregnant woman, family, and
neonate. The team "leader" is not always the physician, as different
problems require different professional expertise. As equal members,
nurses may well find themselves directing the team relative to a problem known best to nursing. This picture is, of course, an ideal;
however, with advanced educational preparation, the nurses are being
more and more accepted by other professionals as equals with a
unique contribution. Nurses, again, need to develop skills necessary to
work successfully with other professionals as equals.

In the field of research, two new forms of research into the
childbearing area involving nurses are emerging: collaborative research and interdisciplinary research. The latter is modeled after the
interdisciplinary team in practice, in that a variety of professionals investigate a problem, each from their own perspective. Collaborative
research, beginning to be found quite often, is a collaboration of a
nurse researcher from an university setting, who presumably directs
the project, and clinical practitioners from the hospital or agency situation, who supply a needed clinical perspective and data-collection site
for the project. Such projects have the potential for great success and

contributions, considering the clinical focus of current research interests and priorities concerning the childbearing family.

SUMMARY

This chapter has provided a brief overview of some trends and issues in the practice of maternal-child health nursing that will affect the nurse. It is, of course, only one perspective. Other interpretations of the same data are possible. The reader is encouraged to read government reports and become aware of state and federal legislation, in order to identify patterns and trends in health care. In this way, the MCH nurse will be a most effective, informed advocate for childbearing families.

REFERENCES

Collins, M, & Natapoff, J. (1984). *A descriptive analysis of maternal and infant health care in New York State.* Report presented to Middle Atlantic Regional Nurses Association and New York State Nurses Association.

Flemming, J. (1985). Maternal-child nursing in the decade ahead. *MCN, The American Journal of Maternal-Child Nursing, 10,* 369–376.

Gartmaker, S. (1979). The effects of prenatal care upon the health of the newborn. *American Journal of Public Health, 69,* 653–657.

Hussey, C., & Scoloveno, M. (1984). A Descriptive Analysis of the Status of Maternal and Infant Care. *Unpublished research.*

March of Dimes Birth Defects Foundation. (1985). *Facts/1985.* White Plains, NY: March of Dimes.

Raff, B. (1984). *Development of core competencies in maternal/infant content in undergraduate nursing education.* Funded Grant Project, U.S. Department of Health and Human Services, Division of Maternal-Child Health Project (MCJ-363510-01-0). Washington, DC.

Index